QUESTIONING
CHEMOTHERAPY

QUESTIONING
CHEMOTHERAPY

RALPH W. MOSS, PH.D.

Equinox Press

Copyright © 1995 by Ralph W. Moss
Manufactured in the United States of America by
Equinox Press
144 St. John's Place
Brooklyn, NY 11217
718-636-4433

Second Printing

Cover and book design by Movable Type, Inc.

Library of Congress Cataloging-in-Publication Data

Moss, Ralph W.
    Questioning chemotherapy / by Ralph W. Moss
        p.   cm.
    Includes bibliographical references and index.
    ISBN 1-881025-25-X
    1. Antineoplastic agents—Side effects.   2. Antineoplastic agents—
Toxicology. 3. Cancer—Chemotherapy—Complications.
4. Antineoplastic agents—Effectiveness. I. Title
RC271.C5M67   1995
616.994 ' 061--dc20   95-11440
                                                                              CIP

Table of Contents

Preface 5

1. Defining Terms 11

2. The Rise of Chemotherapy 15

3. The Profession of Oncology 35

4. The Randomized Clinical Trial 43

5. The Problem of Fraud 53

6. Toxicity of Chemotherapy 67

7. A Multi-Billion-Dollar Business 73

8. Chemo for Particular Cancers 81

9. Quality of Life 151

10. Conclusions 163

Appendix A: Cytotoxic Drugs 171

Appendix B: Some Common Protocols 172

Appendix C: The Major Drugs 173

References 192

Index 210

Preface

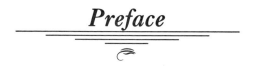

"One may hope that in another 10 to 15 years
medical progress will make this edition of the *Manual of Oncologic
Therapeutics* read like an archaic document for the Middle Ages."
—NCI oncologist Robert E. Wittes, M.D., *Manual of Oncologic Therapeutics* (1991)

"Radical chemotherapy? Unbelievable!
Sounds like the g-ddamned Spanish Inquisition to me."
—"Dr. McCoy" (DeForest Kelley), in *Star Trek IV: The Voyage Home* (1986)

I BEGAN MY CAREER AS A SCIENCE WRITER at Memorial
Sloan-Kettering Cancer Center (MSKCC) in the spring of 1974.
I started out as an enthusiastic believer in chemotherapy. An older
relative had inspired me with the progress he himself had witnessed
during his own medical career. He had "rotated through" Memorial
when he was a doctor in training. In the early 1960s, he recalled, New
York City's famous cancer hospital had to offer interns and residents
lobster dinners just to get them to serve.

By the mid-seventies, when he came to visit me at my new job,
chemotherapy had made significant advances against some forms of
childhood and adolescent cancer, and doctors no longer looked on
childhood leukemia or a dozen other rare types of malignancies as a
death sentence. It was indeed a time of great hope.

The implication of all that I heard and read was that adult cancers
would be the next to fall before this chemical assault. I considered
myself a rationalist, and chemotherapy was "rational therapeutics" par
excellence (66). At MSKCC I thought I had a ringside seat on the
impending cure for cancer and looked forward to doing my own small
bit in helping to bring it about.

As part of my job in the Public Affairs department, I wrote monthly
articles on cancer science for MSKCC's in-house newsletter, *Center
News*. For this, I interviewed many oncologists, often passing through
the hospital's Outpatient Department. I was repeatedly startled by the
sound of unearthly retching coming from the partitioned cubicles.

At first, guided by what these doctors told me, I wrote glowingly
about their triumphs over such rare malignancies as osteogenic sarcoma (bone cancer) and Hodgkin's disease (lymphoma). But I soon
learned about grave reservations that lurked behind even their most

sanguine public pronouncements. Some of the scientists and administrators I encountered intimated—strictly off the record, of course— that finding cures for the common solid tumors of adults, such as breast, colon, and lung, would be an order of magnitude more difficult than treating the unusual pediatric malignancies. In a memorable phrase, one of them told me it would be like trying to dissolve a person's left ear while leaving the right one intact.

I was beginning to feel a vague uneasiness about my role as an ardent promoter of these doctors and their treatments. At the same time, I was proud of my position at MSKCC and determined to do my job well. I had no idea where these vague doubts would eventually lead me.

Some months after I was hired, our department moved from its temporary quarters on East 62nd Street to what was then called the "new hospital" at 68th Street and York Avenue. As part of that move, my boss discarded a collection of handsome departmental scrapbooks that had been gathering dust in a back room. I asked if I could take the binders home to my children, seeing them as ideal for their school reports.

As I began to clean out yellowing newspaper and magazine clippings from the binders, my eye was caught first by one, then another startling story. That summer, almost every evening, I stayed late, systematically reading and saving choice bits of the historical record of Memorial Sloan-Kettering's publicity efforts. I began to augment this with visits to the MSKCC Archives in the hospital basement and to a college library down the block.

A public relations strategy

What I eventually discovered was this: I had been hired to help publicize the latest breakthroughs in the "war on cancer." But publicizing the imminent cure for cancer was nothing new. Rather, for decades it had been the stock-in-trade of newspaper writers, public relations flacks, and "development" (i.e., fund-raising) strategists at Memorial and other medical centers.

At Sloan-Kettering Institute, despite the obligatory lip service to humanitarianism, the focus of some researchers seemed to be a high-paced game of new drug development. The patient, for some of them, was a pawn in the process of discovering and testing new agents that would boost their own careers, and the profits of drug companies.

Money for research was (and continues to be) scarce, no matter how much was pumped into the war on cancer. Scientists therefore sought out pharmaceutical or venture-capital financing. This created an inevitable tendency to try to please their research sponsors.

This impression has been confirmed by a more rigorous survey of clinical trials published in a medical journal. While 61 percent of drug studies in general reported results favorable to a new treatment, for studies supported by pharmaceutical companies the number soared to 89 percent (91). In other words, when the drug company is paying, nine out of ten times scientists find something positive to say, or say nothing at all.

As time went by, I learned that pharmaceutical companies active in the cancer field had assumed positions of great influence on the Board of Overseers (the directorship) of Memorial Sloan-Kettering and its subsidiary corporations. Overseers with fortunes from other sources went into the drug business and became even wealthier. It was a tightening noose.

Bright new minds

Cancer was once seen as a dead end in medicine, and smart doctors hesitated to go into this specialty. But with the creation of the war on cancer, hundreds of millions of dollars were suddenly up for grabs. At around the time that I joined Memorial, cancer research became a smart career move, bringing high salaries, academic prestige, and peer recognition. For a lucky few, it meant really big bucks in the biotech field. Cancer had become big business.

The director of Sloan-Kettering, Robert A. Good, M.D., Ph.D., was famous for speeches extolling the need for fundamental discoveries from "bright new minds." But often the best that profit-oriented scientists at his Institute could come up with were minor modifications of formulas whose patents were running out. This led to boring, incremental change, masquerading as progress. Other scientists were indeed seeking ways to understand the chemical environment of the body (cytokine research, for example). But the practical upshot turned out to be drugs like filgrastim (Neupogen), which enabled clinicians to give increasing amounts of standard toxic chemotherapy to their patients, usually with no appreciable improvement in survival.

Those vague doubts that I experienced more than 20 years ago have now crystallized into the book you hold in your hands. To my knowledge, this is the first book written for the general public in any language that is about the failures as well as the successes of chemotherapy. But it is certainly not the first time trenchant criticisms have emerged. From time to time, researchers have voiced similar reservations within the pages of medical books and journals; but almost never have their qualms been brought to the attention of the general public.

Why such hesitancy? Perhaps it is a fear of damaging long-nurtured careers by appearing disloyal to the cancer establishment. Cancer specialists also sometimes justify their reticence by claiming that a book such as this might discourage people from getting proper medical attention for life-threatening conditions. I doubt that will happen, but let me make my position clear from the start. Namely, there *are* situations where chemotherapy can be a rational and life-saving course. These include most cases of Hodgkin's disease, acute lymphocytic leukemia (ALL), and testicular cancer, as well as certain rare cancers, such as Burkitt's lymphoma, choriocarcinoma, and lymphosarcoma.

It also plays a part, with surgery, in the successful treatment of Wilms' tumor, Ewing's sarcoma, rhabdomyosarcoma, and retinoblastoma.

Among the more common adenocarcinomas, chemotherapy appears to extend survival in many cases of ovarian cancer. In small-cell lung cancer (SCLC) there seems to be a survival gain of several months. Its possible value as an adjuvant treatment in breast cancer patients after potentially curative surgery is discussed at some length below.

Basically, some chemotherapy has its uses; this message will be repeated throughout the text. However, even for the above cancers, chemotherapy remains an often grueling option—medieval, by many doctors' own admission. Even for these kinds of cancer, effective, less-toxic substitutes are therefore still desperately needed.

A reasonable prospect

My point of view in this regard is essentially the same as that of New York cancer specialist, Albert Braverman, M.D., writing in the British medical journal, *The Lancet:*

"Chemotherapy should be prescribed only when there is a reasonable prospect either of cure or of benefit in quantity and quality of life. [O]ncology trainees should be taught that chemotherapy is not part of the management of every cancer patient..." (48).

As I shall explain, for solid tumors of adults, such benefit has rarely been proven and consequently chemotherapy should just as rarely be given.

For reasons of space, our focus shall be only on those three dozen drugs that have been approved by the U.S. Food and Drug Administration (FDA), used either singly or in combinations rather flippantly called "chemo cocktails."

Naturally, this book deals with chemotherapy's record up to this point. Although I personally doubt that cytotoxic drugs (i.e., those that are detrimental or destructive to cells) are about to make any big breakthroughs, admittedly I cannot predict the future. Every new treatment idea certainly deserves to be considered on its own merits, and not rejected because of other drugs' failures.

I am also aware that some doctors use chemotherapy in innovative ways. For example, some doctors use drugs unapproved in their own countries. Others use standard drugs "off-label," for purposes or in dosages that have not been approved by the FDA. This may involve massive doses of conventional drugs.

Some patient advocates, desperate for cures, encourage doctors to pursue even seemingly remote possibilities, such as administering chemotherapy in situations that are unjustified by any scientific results. Even ardent enthusiasts must admit that there is no way to know if such unapproved treatments are really effective. And usually, one doctor's or clinic's astonishing claims of success evaporate when their results are subjected to larger, multi-center studies.

But if such treatments are not subjected to more definitive trials, then these "successes" remain essentially in the realm of anecdote.

It amazes me how much of what passes for knowledge in cancer therapy turns out to be incomplete, inadequate, and anecdotal.

A bitter pill

Early successes with Hodgkin's disease and childhood leukemia stirred up great hopes. As Dr. Braverman points out, some chemotherapists now find it hard to accept the fact that their even greater dreams of curing the common forms of cancer have not come true, and probably never will. That must be a bitter pill indeed. Patients are angry and doctors are defensive; tempers are bound to flair in such a situation. I disagree with almost all the current dogmas of oncology, but do not need to personally attack my opponents in order to build up my own position. Those looking for *ad hominem* attacks will have to look elsewhere.

Chemotherapy's use is now rampant not just in the United States, where it began, but in Canada, Chile, Denmark, France, Germany, Italy, South Africa—actually throughout most of the industrialized, and some of the developing, world. In fact, in Great Britain, 60 different cytotoxic drugs—more than in the United States—are now licensed for use in cancer therapy (61).

With *Questioning Chemotherapy,* I hope to spark an international debate on the value of toxic drugs in the treatment of cancer.

There is much discussion of the meaning of the word "epidemic" in relation to cancer. However, consider this: in 1962, 278,000 Americans died of cancer. By 1982 that figure had risen to over 433,000. By 1995, cancer deaths were estimated at 547,000. Certainly, part of this increase is due to the growth and aging of the population. But even when one adjusts for these, the overall U.S. mortality rate had increased by 10.1 percent from 1950 to 1991 (323). Incidence during that time had increased 49.3 percent. While the occurrence of some cancers declined, many of them were on the rise, sometimes dramatically:

• a 548.7 percent increase in lung cancer among women;

• a 346.7 percent increase in malignant melanoma;

• a 205.4 percent increase in multiple myeloma;

• a 189.9 percent increase in prostate cancer (323).

A sweeping reform of the "war on cancer" is needed, with new leadership focused on prevention, non-invasive forms of early diagnosis, and the exploration of nontoxic and substantially less toxic treatments. A discussion of 102 such approaches is given in my book, *Cancer Therapy* (271).

For the 1.2 million Americans and the 9 million people worldwide (192) who will develop cancer this year, such a reform cannot come too soon.

—R.W.M.

CHAPTER ONE

Defining Terms

DEPENDING ON YOUR POINT OF VIEW, cancer is either the name of more than 100 different conditions, or one condition with many target sites.

Cancer is "a cellular malignancy whose unique trait—loss of normal controls—results in unregulated growth, lack of differentiation, and the ability to invade local tissues and metastasize" (32). The primary growth is usually not fatal. For example, a breast tumor by itself would generally not be a life-threatening condition. Its main danger arises from *metastases*, the spread of the cancer to distant sites and organs, such as the liver, lungs, or brain, as well as from the deleterious effect on the body's metabolism (e.g., a wasting syndrome called *cachexia*).

Metastases are generally what define a case of cancer as *advanced*. And a person with an advanced cancer generally has a much worse prognosis than one whose disease has been caught and treated early.

The word *terminal* is sometimes used to described such advanced patients. It implies that the changes wrought by the cancer are both incurable and irreversible. However, not only do such tumors, against all expectations, occasionally go into spontaneous remission (287), but unexpected "miracle cures" have sometimes been observed following conventional or unconventional treatments (144).

Most experienced doctors have also seen individual patients survive for long periods of time under the most unlikely circumstances. In my opinion, the word terminal and similar words (49) can be a self-fulfilling prophecy and should be banished from the cancer vocabulary.

Types of cancer

Between the vagaries of the tumor, and the variations in treatment, cancer can obviously give rise to a staggering number of individual circumstances.

Cancer is generally divided into broad categories of *neoplasms* (literally, new growths) such as carcinomas, sarcomas, lymphomas, leukemias, and germ cell tumors. Each individual case is classified according to the target organ and the appearance of tissues under the microscope. Here is a quick overview:

Carcinomas are the most common malignancies. They develop in tissues that line the surface of the internal organs and passageways of the body. Most carcinomas develop in an organ that secretes something. For example, the breast secretes milk; the lung, mucus; and the pancreas, digestive juices. Carcinomas include, among others, most of the malignant tumors of the trachea, lung, stomach, colon, rectum, esophagus, breast, bladder, pancreas, ovary, cervix, head and neck, and liver. Since their linings are epithelial tissues, carcinomas are also sometimes called epithelial cancers or *epitheliomas*. Carcinomas cause over 80 percent of the cancer deaths in the industrialized world.

Sarcomas are cancers of the connective tissue. They generally start either in the bone or cartilage, fat, connective tissue, or muscle. There are nearly two dozen different kinds of sarcomas. They are more common in children than adults.

Germ cell tumors mainly arise in the testes. While a relatively rare kind of cancer, these are the most common cancers in men between the ages of 15 and 34, a time of life when cancer is uncommon.

*Leukemia*s are cancers of the blood cells (leukocytes). They most commonly involve a wild proliferation of immature white blood cells.

Lymphomas are cancers of the lymphoid system. These are divided into two main types: Hodgkin's disease, named after a nineteenth century physician, and non-Hodgkin's lymphomas, which are about five times as common as Hodgkin's disease.

Multiple myeloma is another disease of the blood system, characterized by the proliferation of the antibody-producing B lymphocytes.

Malignant melanomas are cancers of the pigment-producing cells called melanocytes. They generally start as a mole, which begins to grow and can then metastasize (spread) throughout the entire body.

The staging of cancer

Among the first things an oncologist (cancer specialist) will generally do is to "stage" the tumor. This conveys to other doctors how far advanced the case is, and helps to determine both the prognosis (the course the disease is likely to take) and the most likely treatment.

There is a widely adopted international system for categorizing cases of cancer, called the TNM system. This describes each individual case of cancer by the size of the tumor (T), the involvement of regional lymph nodes (N), and the extent of distant metastases (M), if any.

TNM designations can get complicated. In breast cancer, for instance, there are five different Ts, four Ns, and three Ms, which can occur in various combinations.

Doctors also refer to the spread of the disease by the older Roman numeral stages of severity. According to this way of grading cases, there are seven different and distinct stages of breast cancer—stage 0, stage I, stage IIA, stage IIB, stage IIIA, stage IIIB, and stage IV. Not all cancer staging conforms to the TNM system. Thus, colon cancer is generally referred to by the Dukes' classification system, while small-cell lung cancer is designated as either limited or extensive. Certain tumors of the female reproductive tract are designated by an international gynecological organization's "FIGO" staging system. Melanomas are often classed via the Clark or Breslow classifications for the depth of invasion of the tumor.

Prognoses are averages

Staging is important in making a prognosis of the patient's case. Remember, however, that such prognoses are essentially averages, and in no sense should be taken as an iron rule for individual cases. It is hard to escape the impression, however, that for some patients the prognosis becomes a self-fulfilling prophecy, and they almost feel required to die on schedule, as predicted by their doctors. Doctors are sometimes very unfeeling in making such predictions. Patients and family members should clearly understand that there is nothing inevitable about such numbers. Every case is unique.

What are relapses?

It is also important to grasp the concept of the relapse, for it explains much about the failures in chemotherapy. The goal of chemotherapy is to poison cancer cells in the body. But tumors have the ability to develop a resistance to the assault of cytotoxic drugs. Often, after an apparently successful treatment, the cancer will return.

Anyone who has ever fought insects with pest sprays understands the rudiments of such "population genetics." The susceptible ones die off, while the hearty and resistant ones survive and thrive. Malignant cells as a community also naturally resist being wiped out. As part of their own struggle for survival, they can develop biochemical resistance to cytotoxic drugs.

Oncologists attempt to overcome what is called the clinical resistance of the patient, generally by attempting to make all cancer cells divide on cue. This is called synchronizing the growth cycles of the cancer cells. However, despite many efforts in this direction, so far tumor cells have been able to develop resistance to all existing cytotoxic drugs. That is one reason that tumors frequently grow back rapidly after chemotherapy. It is also part of the reason that once a relapse occurs, a second complete remission with conventional drugs is extremely rare.

Curative chemotherapy

The primary goal of curative chemotherapy is to kill every last cancer cell lurking in the body. Its method is to shrink and destroy the primary cancer and all measurable metastases, and by doing so to bring about disease-free periods of remissions that are so lengthy that the patient will live out his or her normal life span. As we shall show, this goal involves a number of unproven hypotheses, and has been nearly impossible to attain in most kinds of cancer.

Some other uses of chemotherapy

For that reason, a number of other goals are also pursued through the use of chemotherapy.

Induction treatment This is the use of cytotoxic drugs to first reduce the size and extent of locally advanced tumors so that surgery and/or radiation can more efficiently do their work. For example, when a woman has a very large and extensive primary breast tumor, doctors will often give her chemotherapy first in order to bring about "clear margins" for a later operation.

Induction therapy has sometimes yielded high "response rates," such as in head and neck cancer. Because of this apparent success, for years chemotherapists hailed induction therapy as a coming triumph for their methods. After many clinical trials, however, the concept has fallen far short of the hopes invested in it.

Adjuvant treatment After potentially curative surgery, patients are still in danger of a relapse. To try and wipe out little nests of "micrometastases," doctors may give chemotherapy to symptom-free patients after their surgery, to reduce the chance of a recurrence. Although such adjuvant treatment has been tried in many kinds of cancers, it is most commonly used today in women after surgery for breast cancer and in patients with regionally spread colon cancer.

Palliative treatment Chemotherapy can be given to shrink disfiguring or painful tumors, especially those that are externally visible. Such use is appropriate in a small minority of cases. But chemotherapy is often given to palliate cancer or improve the quality of life in many other cases. Does it really do so, or does it further weaken and endanger the patient? We shall discuss the successes and failures of both adjuvant and palliative therapy in the chapters that follow.

CHAPTER TWO

The Rise of Chemotherapy

THE USE OF CHEMICALS IN CANCER goes back at least to the time of Paracelsus (1493-1541), sometimes called the "father of chemotherapy." In the nineteenth and early twentieth century, arsenic in the form of Fowler's solution was administered to patients (125); caustic chemicals, such as zinc chloride, were rubbed onto external tumors; poisonous lead was injected into women as a treatment for advanced breast cancer (292); and benzene was employed against leukemia—an odd choice, since benzene is now known to cause leukemia (325).

The word "chemotherapy" essentially means the use of chemicals in the treatment of disease. It was coined in 1907 by Nobel laureate Paul Ehrlich (1854-1915), whose main work was the treatment of venereal diseases. In 1909, he formulated his famous Salvarsan 606, a drug injected intravenously for the treatment of syphilis. This was hailed at the time as a "new science" of drug use. It was not auspicious, however, that by 1914, 109 deaths had been attributed to this arsenic-containing compound (389). An American doctor of the time noted, "Even the poor can scarcely be expected to submit with good grace to repeated barbarities offered in the name of medicine" (357).

Undeterred, Ehrlich turned his attention to cancer. In fact, he himself was among the first to describe the effects of so-called *alkylating agents* on cells and organs, presaging their later use against cancer (111,148).

With increasing frequency, the term *chemotherapy*, or as it is popularly abbreviated *chemo*, has come to refer specifically to the chemical treatment of malignant (cancerous) diseases. It was the same Paul Ehrlich who also coined the memorable phrase "magic bullet," to refer to a hypothetical drug that could act with the specificity of natural antibodies. This magic bullet, sometimes confused with the Lone Ranger's silver projectile, became the shimmering goal of chemotherapy.

"[T]he chemotherapists of the new century brought a special zeal to their cause," wrote Brown University historian James T. Patterson. "They believed their magic bullets would be the salvation of humanity" (295). From the start, however, cancer chemotherapy "proved deeply disappointing." The new drugs had "little effect" and were often highly toxic, killing "mice and rats as fast as or faster

15

than the cancers" (295).

For that reason, practicing physicians were deeply skeptical of the whole idea of what they called "constitutional" remedies. Sloan-Kettering researcher Kanematsu Sugiura, D.Sc., a pioneer of experimental cancer chemotherapy, once told me that in the 1920s chemotherapists were looked upon as little better than quacks. And according to Alfred Gilman, Ph.D., another founder, "[I]n the minds of most physicians the administration of drugs, other than an analgesic, in the treatment of malignant disease was the act of a charlatan" (140).

It is amusing to read how surgeons and radiologists of the 1930s used exactly the same arguments against those who employed such "constitutional" agents as the chemotherapists of today use against "alternative" doctors (87,292).

The mustard gas experiments

The modern era of chemotherapy is often dated from December, 1943 with the explosion of an Allied Liberty ship, the *John E. Harvey*, in the harbor of Bari, Italy (193). The ship was laden with poisonous mustard gas, similar to that which had been used with devastating effectiveness in World War I. Sailors who survived the Bari explosion later suffered from a severe depression of their bone marrow, and some of them even died from a near-complete depletion of white blood cells. This anomaly was astutely described by a Navy doctor, Peter Alexander.

Unknown to Dr. Alexander, however, animal and even clinical (human) trials of mustard gas derivatives were already under way "under the cloak of war-time secrecy" (342) at Yale University by the time the *John E. Harvey* exploded. And in fact it had long been known that mustard gas was harmful to the blood-making system (218). Scientists at Memorial Hospital had even applied a form of mustard gas externally to breast cancer lesions in the 1930s (6).

Chemical warfare experiments

In early 1942, the U.S. government had signed a contract with Yale University and other research centers to generally investigate chemical warfare agents. There was in fact an informal network of such secret laboratories across the U.S. The Nazis were working on a similar class of agents (318), and the British also had their own program (148).

For experimental purposes at Yale a nitrogen atom had been substituted for a sulfur atom in the mustard gas, yielding a liquid compound, soluble in water or alcohol, which was called "nitrogen mustard."

Tissues susceptible to the effects of nitrogen mustard, wrote Gilman, "were those with renewal cell populations, primarily lymphoid tissue, bone marrow and the epithelium of the gastrointestinal tract" (140).

It was Dr. Thomas Dougherty, a Yale anatomist, who is credited with the idea of injecting this nitrogen mustard into mice with tumors. He chose an animal which had been injected with lymphoma cells that formed a huge tumor. The life span of such an animal following the transplantation of cancer cells was usually about three weeks.

One lone mouse

"We gave [nitrogen] mustard to this one lone mouse which had a fairly advanced tumor," Dougherty recalled. "After just two administrations of the compound the tumor began to soften and regress."

But in one month, the tumor recurred. "We then treated the animal again and a regression occurred again, although it was not as complete as the first time," he added. In all, the animal lived 84 days—"a very remarkable prolongation of survival," Dougherty called it.

Other experiments quickly followed, in as many strains of rodents as were then available. Yet, oddly, Yale scientists were unable to duplicate the success of that first mouse. They didn't even come close.

"The only one of the murine [mouse, ed.] lymphomas in which we got complete regression was in the original tumor in which we tried the compound," Dougherty remembered (140). "The very first mouse treated turned out to give the best result....In most of the murine leukemias, particularly those which metastasize readily, we frequently obtained no effect at all."

He added: "I have often thought that if we had by accident chosen one of these leukemias...we might possibly have dropped the whole project" (140).

Compound X

Nevertheless, based essentially on success in this solitary mouse, human clinical trials were initiated in early December, 1942 on a patient in the advanced stages of lymphosarcoma, a diffuse form of lymphoma.

"The selection of a proper dose of a highly toxic chemical warfare agent for administration to man for the first time," Gilman recalled, "was made with unwarranted confidence." There was a great deal of mystery surrounding the experiment. The entry on the patient's chart read, "0.1 mg per kg compound X given intravenously" and everything to do with the treatment was classified "top secret."

Gilman reported that "the response of the first patient was as dramatic as the first mouse." The man's tumor masses softened within 48 hours and obstructive signs and symptoms were relieved within 10 days. Huge lymph nodes in his armpits completely disappeared. The scientists were euphoric; here was "heroic medicine" indeed! But there was trouble on the horizon. Within four weeks the patient's white blood cell count plummeted from 5,000 per cubic millimeter to around 200. He developed severe clotting problems. The tumor then "regenerated with the bone marrow—a great disappointment," said Gilman. Subsequent courses of treatment resulted in only transient improvement, and the man died.

Trials and tribulations

"Twenty years later," Gilman wrote in 1959, "we can appreciate how accurately this first patient reflected the future trials and tribulations of therapy with alkylating agents." And indeed, "almost without exception," according to two authors of a medical textbook on toxicity, "every drug developed for four decades that is active against cancer has produced side effects that are reminiscent of the outgrowth of these agents from research on chemical warfare" (298).

The next patient treated suffered the same destruction of his bone marrow but without a "concomitant clinical response." Five more patients with a variety of tumors were treated at Yale. Reading between the lines, we gather that here too the treatment was a failure. (Their cases "serve to point out the limitations of therapy with the nitrogen mustards," is how Gilman tactfully put it.)

But nitrogen mustard was "the first synthetic compound clearly shown to possess anti-tumor activity in humans" (177) and scientists were extremely excited by this finding. In June 1943, the nitrogen mustard group at Yale dispersed, but they disseminated their excitement about their top secret results to colleagues at the University of Chicago, within the U.S. military, and elsewhere. In all, it is said that 160 patients received chemotherapy in this period. But there were no reported cures.

The era of Farber and Rhoads

The leader of the U.S. Army Chemical Warfare Service at that time was Cornelius P. "Dusty" Rhoads (1898-1959), then a rising star of cancer research. Rhoads had been a Rockefeller Foundation fellow, and had been at Memorial Hospital. After the war, he was chosen as the first head of the newly formed Sloan-Kettering Institute for Cancer Research, the research arm of what became Memorial Sloan-Kettering Cancer Center (269). In 1940, he had spelled out his own philosophy in a speech to a group of patent attorneys:

"In the near future patents may well control its [medicine's] entire development," he said. "The patent lawyers can and do control the support of industrial science. I wish to establish clearly the need for, as well as the profits to be obtained from, intelligent study of the factors which influence the course of illness" (319).

In the post-war period, Rhoads launched a vigorous program of drug experimentation. He "was absolutely determined that the cure for cancer was going to be found in his institute and nowhere else," one reporter remembered (145). He became an effective "evangelist of chemotherapy," wrote Patterson (295). On June 27, 1949, Rhoads and his new Institute were even featured on the cover of *Time* magazine.

Dr. Sidney Farber of Boston was another tireless innovator and promoter of chemotherapy. He is credited with the discovery of "antimetabolites" and brought about the first temporary remissions in childhood leukemia. Other hormonal drugs, such as ACTH and cortisone, were also brought to bear. What Sloan-Kettering's David Karnofsky called the "golden age of chemotherapy" was being born (205).

Chemical marvels

In retrospect, "the interest in cancer chemotherapy was part of a broader, post-war fascination with chemical marvels," according to Patterson (295). With the introduction of "sulfa" drugs (sulfonamides), medicine began to emerge "from a period of therapeutic nihilism," in which all new agents were suspect (140). The success of penicillin and streptomycin were major inspirations for this effort. In fact, penicillin "was already clearing out the pediatric wards of hospitals, freeing doctors to experiment with drugs on leukemia victims" (295). In 1953, Rhoads enthused, "Inevitably, as I see it, we can look forward to something like a penicillin for cancer, and I hope within the next decade" (295).

The nothing-is-too-stupid-to-test program

There was also a fascination with the "big science" approach to solving urgent national problems. The parallels with the Manhattan Project that produced the atomic bomb were clear. It was assumed that the anticipated "magic bullet" would come from Sloan-Kettering Institute, the National Cancer Institute (NCI), or the Ivy League medical schools. More than one young chemotherapist fancied himself the Louis Pasteur of cancer.

In this period, Sloan-Kettering and the NCI examined over 400,000 chemicals as potential drugs; 10,000 new ones are still added every year (177). About two thousand have been reported "to have selective toxicity for at least one kind of tumor cells" (177) and eventually these yielded about 50 items destructive of cancer. These drugs are still the backbone of what is called the cytotoxic "armamentarium." Some skeptics called this the "nothing-is-too-stupid-to-test" program and observed "that chemical testing enriched pharmaceutical companies that patented the drugs" (295).

No intellectual appeal

Not everyone was swept up in this early enthusiasm for chemotherapy, however. A director of the NCI itself, Kenneth M. Endicott, was initially unconvinced, recalling "we really didn't have the necessary information to engineer a program...it was premature, and well, it just had no intellectual appeal to me whatever" (114).

To hear chemotherapists tell it, in those days they were a beleaguered minority group within medicine. "The medical community had strong reservations about the method and its practitioners," wrote chemotherapist (turned critic) Albert Braverman, M.D. (48). Some scientists recoiled at the horrendous toxicity they were beginning to see. Patients were retching, their hair was falling out, and they were dying from drug-related destruction of their bone marrow. Agents with side effects such as these had not been seen since the days of high-dose calomel (mercurous chloride) in previous centuries. It was supposed to be a thing of the past.

"The mere word 'chemotherapy' causes an attack of gastric acidity and a sudden rise in blood pressure in many physicians who consider it a dangerous—nay, diabolical—weapon," French oncologist Lucien Israel wrote (193).

The battle simmers

This battle within the medical profession simmered for decades. But the skeptics of the time were fighting a rear-guard action, as boosters ratcheted up their rhetoric, buoyed by longer and longer remissions in childhood leukemia and Hodgkin's disease, and encouraged by a growing pharmaceutical interest.

Sidney Farber called the chemo effort "the greatest mobilization of resources...ever undertaken to conquer a single disease." Rhoads enthused, "it is no longer a question if cancer will be controlled, but when and how soon."

The scientific director of the ardently pro-chemotherapy American Cancer Society (ACS), Dr. Charles Cameron, traveled the country with two hamsters given to him by Farber. These were presented at meetings as living proof of the wonders of the chemical "cure."

Even the once-skeptical Endicott was finally converted, and chimed in with such statements as "the next step—the complete cure—is almost sure to follow" (295).

Penicillin for cancer?

"I am convinced that in the next decade, or maybe more, we will have a chemical as effective against cancer as sulfanilamide and penicillin are against bacterial infection," Rhoads told the *Denver Post* (10/3/53).

"There is, for the first time, a scent of ultimate victory in the air," read an article on cytotoxic drugs in *Reader's Digest* in February, 1957.

"Nothing short of spectacular...a work of monumental importance," is how a New York chemotherapist described some now forgotten drug treatment for breast cancer in 1976 in the N.Y. *Daily News* (2/17/76).

The rhetoric had no bounds, as chemotherapists ensconced themselves at the National Cancer Institute and in the major hospitals across the country. They sensed ultimate victory in the air. And indeed, the results in childhood leukemia and Hodgkin's disease led many to believe that they would soon deliver on their promises.

A hopeful fervor

By the late 1960s it seemed as if the whole world was in a "hopeful fervor" (160) over the impending cure. Dr. R. Lee Clark, director of the M.D. Anderson Hospital and Tumor Institute in Houston, told a committee of the U.S. Congress that "with a billion dollars a year for ten years we could lick cancer" (269).

It was a grand illusion, as many on the inside knew, but it soon led to the greatest expenditure of money for biomedical research in world history. On December 23, 1971, the "war on cancer" was launched—President Nixon's "Christmas present to the nation."

"Today," Lucien Israel wrote in the mid-1970s, "one has only to open the *Cancer Treatment Reports* published regularly by the U.S. National Cancer Institute to realize that...the cause of polychemotherapies has definitely triumphed..." (193). About critics, he remarked with cool disdain, "The dogs bark, but the caravan moves on" (193).

Israel's popular book, *Conquering Cancer,* is filled with the aggressive, crusading optimism of those days. A few quotations will give the flavor.

The drawbacks of chemotherapy "have largely disappeared," he wrote. "I fail to understand how one can justify abstaining from treatment....Chemotherapy is no longer the difficult, toxic treatment it was ten years ago....[T]he next few years will see the emergence of an arsenal of new drugs which...will be increasingly effective..." (193).

21

Dominant subspecialty

Chemotherapeutic agents were clearly dangerous; this danger called into existence highly trained experts, such as oncologists/hematologists and chemotherapists. Oncology nurses and technicians had to be trained to deal with potentially deadly drugs and regimens. Specialized government-sanctioned comprehensive cancer centers had to be built and staffed. In a few decades, oncologists went from being a minor group within the profession to an important, even dominant, subspecialty of medicine.

Today's oncologist provides a dazzling display of medical skill, as he or she manipulates huge amounts of knowledge of the actions and interactions of literally scores of toxic compounds.

"The consequences of an error in dosage or dose adjustment may be lethal," warned Dr. Bruce Chabner, former Director of the Division of Cancer Treatment at the National Cancer Institute (66). This is strong medicine. It is the job of the oncologists to guard the portals of existence itself, to guide the patient to the "vital frontier," i.e., the very brink of death, and then hopefully back again.

But sometimes they fail. In December, 1994, Betsy Lehman, health columnist for the *Boston Globe,* died when Dana-Farber Cancer Institute doctors gave her a four-fold overdose of the drug cyclophosphamide. At least a dozen doctors, nurses, and pharmacists failed to detect the error, and it then escaped attention for four months. "Doctors apparently refused to heed her warnings that something was drastically wrong and ignored the results of tests indicating heart damage," Dr. Lawrence K. Altman wrote in the *New York Times* (3/24/95).

A military tone

Irwin D. Bross, Ph.D., former Director of Biostatistics at New York State's Roswell Park Memorial Institute for Cancer Research, has remarked on the "macho" nature of the profession of oncology. Perhaps it was its origin in World War II that gave rise to this mentality.

The overriding metaphor is, of course, that of a "war" against cancer. We have now become accustomed to talk of "weapons," "strategies," and a whole "armamentarium" of cell-killing drugs. Combinations of drugs bear aggressive-sounding acronyms like BOLD, CHOP, COP, COP-BLAM, ICE, MOP, and ProMACE. Oncologists are the "soldiers on the front lines" with "armor forged for them in medical school" (193).

This military language has become so ingrained that it is difficult to even talk about cancer without resorting to war images. Although patients may feel reassured to hear their doctors talking tough about cancer, this mind-set has not taken us very far in the last 50 years, and is not likely to do so in the future.

As University of Manitoba oncologist Harvey Schipper, M.D. has pointed out, "Experimentation procedures, evaluation criteria, and therapies are all based on cell killing. Yet there is substantial evidence that the kill/cure paradigm has reached its limit, and may be blinding us to other mechanisms to control this family of diseases" (335).

Brute force strategies

"Why are brute force strategies so popular?" asked Irwin Bross. "The 'heroic' chemotherapists discovered an easy way to make a big reputation for 'research' overnight. Their strategy was to be more macho than their more cautious colleagues: simply increase the dosage past the point of prudence. If the strategy failed, the mistakes were buried; if it happened to succeed, the chemotherapist could be an instant 'hero' and publish a lot of papers" (55). Failures could be conveniently ascribed to an insufficient dose of the poisons.

The rationale for all this misguided activity was the prevalent doctrine that to be successful doctors had "to kill every last tumor cell." But to achieve this chimeral dream, doctors would in fact need to "destroy the patient's host defense system long before that goal was achieved"—to "destroy the village in order to save it," to use an analogy from the Vietnam war.

Yet "despite (or perhaps because of) its inherent absurdities, 'heroic chemotherapy' became the dominant U.S. doctrine for cancer therapy," Bross concluded (55).

The media connection

Since the 1940s, an interlocking cancer establishment of top hospitals, research centers, government and private agencies, and regulatory bodies, have held sway over the public's perception of cancer (269). What little criticism there has been remained buried deep in the pages of medical journals (117,254,288). But the selling of chemotherapy was not easy, and could never have been accomplished without a compliant media. How did that happen?

Fine and friendly relations

Starting in the 1930s, a new kind of journalist emerged, the science writer. These specialists established collegial relationships with their sources. In a speech to a large science convention in 1936, David Dietz, an early president of the National Association of Science Writers (NASW), spoke of the "fine and friendly relations which now exist between the scientists and the press." At press conferences, for instance, scientists were allowed to dodge impromptu interrogation and submit their own written questions in advance of the interview. Reporters were convinced to first "check their impressions" with "competent and responsible authorities." Scientists were assured that they would be treated with "dignity" and "respect," and with "no distortion of emphasis" or "unfair implications" placed on their work (101).

In exchange for better access for a few, the typical pencil-behind-the-ear reporter was no longer allowed to harry dignified scientists with unseemly questions. This arrangement eliminated some of the vulgarization of science, to be sure. But it is easy to see how such a cozy compact could—and did—result in the manipulation of the press by scientists and public relations experts with axes to grind.

Perky cheerleaders

"We science journalists...too often serve as perky cheerleaders for our subject and our sources," *New York Times* writer Natalie Angier observed in 1991. "We sometimes end up writing copy that sounds like an unvarnished press release" (14).

Editors and presumably readers wanted to hear good news, not gloomy exposés of failure. Thus, like the scientists, journalists had a "publication bias" of their own: a strong incentive to subscribe to a gospel of success about cancer and to ignore negative findings. A study in the *Journal of the American Medical Association* has shown that when reporters were given both positive and negative stories on a new drug, about half of them chose to write *only* about the positive findings; and none of them chose to write solely about the negative results (212).

We ourselves conducted an on-line search of the coverage of chemotherapy by the *Chicago Tribune* between the years 1988 to 1995. We chose the "Trib" because of its excellent record in exposing the coverup of fraud in the breast cancer trials in 1994. However, our search turned up few stories critical of chemotherapy. Instead, we found scores of laudatory articles with headlines such as:

- "Chemotherapy Plus Surgery Increase Odds in Lung Cases"
- "High Cure Rate Reported in Chemotherapy Test"
- "Chemo Can Be Lifesaver, If You Can Stand It"
- "Breast Cancer Drugs Can Add Years of Life"
- "Newest Research Confirms Hope in Fight Against Cancer"
- "Experts Zero in on 'Magic Bullet' to Kill Cancer Cells"

For decades, enthusiastic writers, following the lead of chemo-therapy's promoters, have lauded the latest "magic bullet" treatment for the disease. Rarely has a writer revisited a story to see if a promised cancer "cure"actually panned out.

Oncologists to the rescue!

Any sign of disaffection has been quickly rejoined by vigilant scientists, grateful patients, or media watchdogs.

One example: in 1991, Julia Roberts and Campbell Scott starred in a movie called "Dying Young." The movie was a box-office flop, but did manage to depict some of the realities of one person's struggle with cancer. It showed a wealthy young man undergoing treatment for acute leukemia. He vomits, feels socially isolated by the disease, and finally abandons his treatment.

Oncologists to the rescue! In an article entitled "Experts Fear Movie May Perpetuate Misconceptions about Chemotherapy," Dr. Ronald Blum, head of New York University's Cancer Center, explained that such side effects are virtually a thing of the past. The Blum interview was (and is) circulated by *The Cancer Weekly* on the Compuserve computer network.

Side effects are minimal

"A recent and dramatic medical advance—a new type of drug called Zofran (ondansetron HCl)," Dr. Blum said, "can prevent chemo-therapy-induced emesis [vomiting, ed.] in most cancer patients, even those receiving very toxic cytotoxic drugs. Moreover," he said, "side effects of the medicine are minimal and easily managed. Among the most common are headache, treatable with over-the-counter anal-gesics, and diarrhea."

In truth, ondansetron may be a valuable drug for people undergoing chemotherapy. But four years later, it is still essentially unproven. It is certainly more expensive than the drugs that it would replace and some of the papers (201) and newspaper articles (18) reporting its benefits originate with this patented drug's manufacturer, a subsidiary of Glaxo, Inc.

Sacred cow

For the media, chemotherapy is a sacred cow. When it is even mildly criticized, as it was by implication in this movie, defenders will do or say almost anything to keep the public convinced of its value.

The taming of the natural skepticism of the press was not achieved easily. In cancer, it was mainly set in motion by the American Cancer

Society and its founding power brokers, Mary and Albert Lasker and Elmer Bobst. They had vast experience in this sort of thing. Lasker was a superb advertising man and publicist, who among other things thought up the advertising campaign for Lucky Strikes cigarettes. For many years, Mrs. Lasker presided over the Lasker Awards, a kind of American training ground for Nobel laureates. Bobst was president of several major drug companies with interests in the cancer field.

Hope and fear

As an historian of the American Cancer Society (ACS) once wrote: "From the beginning it vacillated between a fear technique and the dissemination of hope" (63). The ACS needn't have vacillated, since both approaches worked well in tandem, and it has become among the largest fund-raising agencies in the world (31).

On the one hand, they played on the public's growing fear of cancer. "Cancer Kills People" was the theme of the 1945 campaign, complete with pictures of coffins and gravestones.

"One in five of us here—every fifth person in the audience—will get cancer," Bobst would intone at public meetings (40). (Today, it is one in three.) This helped engender cancer-phobia in the general public, a free-floating anxiety that was then relieved by the good news of impending drug breakthroughs. This approach worked well. From the first time it was tried out in *Reader's Digest* in late 1944, the modern approach to cancer fund raising stimulated millions of dollars in donations and provided political support for a billion-dollar crash program to cure cancer.

The barrage of cancer stories in the media was (and remains) unrelenting. In one 40-day period in 1981, NCI counted 1,500 newspaper and magazine articles about cancer (324). A computerized search for the word "cancer" turned up over 23,000 references in the pages of the *Los Angeles Times* alone in the decade between 1985 and 1995. As reporter Daniel Greenberg suggested, much of this ultimately originates in the public affairs departments of the cancer industry itself (156).

Cancer month

Typically these stories reach a crescendo in April, which is the officially designated "cancer month" in the United States. It was on April 25, 1994 that *Time* magazine's cover blared out in red letters two inches high, "Hope in the War Against Cancer."

Later that year, the Scripps Research Institute in La Jolla, California issued a press release that an experimental drug had shown promise in chicken eggs, not even rats or mice. But the Scripps news release claimed: "This approach not only is expected to eliminate primary tumors but also will likely prevent the metastatic spread of tumor cells by eliminating their access to the blood supply."

A "giant leap of faith," is how Lawrence K. Altman, M.D. later described it in the *New York Times* (1/10/95), laying blame at the feet of medical press agents. But even the *Times* itself ran the story on its front page, and it was highlighted on network news shows that evening.

As Dr. Martin Shapiro of the University of California at Los Angeles has said, "Cancer researchers, medical journals and the popular media all have contributed to a situation in which many people with common malignancies are being treated with drugs not known to be effective."

Yet, he added, "The public needs to be skeptical of purveyors of allegedly effective treatments for these cancers." The media in particular should "stop proclaiming every report on a new cancer drug as the breakthrough that could emancipate humankind from malignancy" (340).

But this is unlikely to happen, because proclaiming the imminent cure for cancer is as good for the media business as it is for the chemotherapy business.

The glory years

In the decades between 1960 and 1980, chemotherapists generally enjoyed a grace period during which the public ardently believed that a cure for cancer was around the corner. By 1971, 25 different drugs were already in use against cancer. These included not just nitrogen mustard, but such commonly used drugs as cyclophosphamide, methotrexate, fluorouracil (5-FU), vincristine, and BCNU (408).

The cure for cancer became part of the national mythology. To use the language of sociology, it was given "a special place in the commercially organized fantasies of the nation" (146). Like any profession, oncology now had its "cant or pose" which had the effect "of a conspiracy to work upon the credulity of the rest of the world" (82). Of course, there had to be some basis in fact, no matter how small, for such a widely held belief.

It was during this period that chemotherapy was shown to cause long-term remissions in relatively rare, but certainly tragic forms of cancer in children, such as acute lymphocytic leukemia, as well as in a disease of young adults, Hodgkin's disease. In addition, as we have pointed out, chemotherapy also contributed to the successful treatment of almost a dozen other rare kinds of cancer such as Burkitt's lymphoma, choriocarcinoma, lymphosarcoma, Wilms' tumor, Ewing's sarcoma, rhabdomyosarcoma, and retinoblastoma.

The seventies also saw the first successful treatment of embryonal testicular cancer with the then-new platinum-based compounds. It was largely based on what seemed to be a cascade of successes that the war on cancer was launched. There was a widespread belief that solid tumors would be the next to fall before the same chemical onslaught.

Experience in treating childhood cancers led to escalating dosages of drugs in an attempt to bring about complete remissions, and of increasingly complicated combinations, to overcome clinical resistance.

"With suitable combinations of chemicals it is now possible to cure many kinds of childhood cancer that would otherwise be rapidly fatal," John Cairns, Professor of Microbiology at the Harvard University School of Public Health, said in 1985 (60). Although a minority of patients relapsed and died during or soon after ending their course of therapy, many others went on to prolonged periods of relapse-free survival.

This success could be seen in the mortality statistics. In the early 1950s, about 1,900 children under the age of five died of cancer each year. By the 1980s, this had fallen to about 700 each year. About two-thirds of all children with cancer were therefore being "cured."

Among young adults, the results were less spectacular, with the notable exception of Hodgkin's disease. This had been an almost invariably fatal illness, but with cytotoxic drugs (and/or radiotherapy) it was almost routinely put into long-term remission. This represented a savings of about 1,000 lives each year in the U.S.

Testicular cancer also had been almost invariably fatal. When Cairns wrote, about 35 percent of such patients were being saved by chemotherapy, for a total savings of about 300 lives per year.

Finally, choriocarcinoma, a rare cancer of pregnancy, was controlled through the use of drugs, such as methotrexate. In the U.S., this represented a savings of another 20 to 30 lives per year.

Successful treatments

For the people involved, of course, these successful treatments were remarkable. Many of us are old enough to remember when Hodgkin's disease and childhood leukemia were virtual death sentences. By comparison, many of us now know people with these diseases whose lives have been extended or saved by chemotherapy.

In 1985, there were about 7,000 deaths per year from cancer in those under the age of 30. One would have expected 10,000 to die if the death rate had remained unchanged since the 1950s. Thus, there was a savings of 3,000 lives. However, one must put these successes into the context of the overall cancer tragedy. This occurred in a country where every year cancer kills over half a million people.

"Only two percent of the patients who die of cancer are under 30," Cairns cautioned, and this figure has changed little in the intervening decade. "For the vast majority of cancers, which arise in older patients, the results of chemotherapy are much more controversial"(60).

As soon as efforts were made to extend such punishing treatments to older patients, however, serious problems emerged. The amount of toxic chemicals needed to kill every last cancer cell was found to kill the patient long before it eliminated the tumor. When doctors tried such high-dose treatments they created societal resistance to what was seen as a reversion to the barbaric treatments of the Middle Ages.

Pockets of resistance

Although the cancer establishment generally held sway over both public and scientific opinion, this was not without notable pockets of resistance. During this period, a few souls within the biomedical community have dared to criticize the direction of cancer research. Almost always, they have limited their complaints to medical and scientific publications, and their arguments never reached the general public.

For a period of time in the mid-1970s, Nobel laureate James Watson, one of the world's most respected biologists, repeatedly called the war on cancer scientifically bankrupt, therapeutically ineffective, and wasteful (156). In March 1975, he was quoted as saying that the American public had been "sold a nasty bill of goods about cancer" (*New York Times*, 3/9/75).

In 1975, reporter Daniel S. Greenberg broke a virtual media blockade with a celebrated piece in the *Columbia Journalism Review (CJR)* (155). This was the first time that a respected journalist had dared to openly criticize the cancer establishment. The January/February 1975 *CJR* article quoted many criticisms by oncologists and statisticians working within the "war" itself. In March, Greenberg wrote a follow-up article for the *New England Journal of Medicine* (156). Both articles showed that claims of progress were a sham, a statistical construct.

For me and many of my colleagues, the Greenberg affair was an eye-opener. I remember how copies of his articles were excitedly passed from hand to hand in our office. It confirmed our own latent suspicions that the "war on cancer" was fundamentally flawed.

Gullible reporters

Greenberg claimed that "the lay press" was "unduly gullible in reporting 'progress' in cancer treatment." He showed that claims of vastly improved cancer rates were highly exaggerated. Survival rates had changed little for the types of cancer that "account for 78 percent of the incidence of the disease." In fact, there was an actual decline in survival rates for cancers that account for approximately 13 percent of incidence.

Greenberg compared the statements of the cancer warriors to the "light-at-the-end-of-the-tunnel" thesis of the then-fresh Vietnam war. Most of his quotations, however, were from anonymous statisticians, and he was taunted for this by an American Cancer Society spokesperson. Anonymity was necessary, he explained, since many cancer scientists were afraid to speak out publicly.

Greenberg recalled how one senior scientist told him, "The official line is that we're making a lot of progress....It just doesn't pay to rock the boat." He concluded, "The vast and ill-conceived undertaking that was created by the National Cancer Act of 1971 has inevitably spawned a monolithic bureaucracy with a heavily supported public-relations apparatus that is simply misleading the American public on a dreadfully serious subject" (156). For me personally, Greenberg's acerbic remarks about "public relations" certainly hit home.

The politics of cancer

In 1976, the well-known social critic Ivan Illich published his influential *Medical Nemesis*, a still-relevant book about the scope of doctor-caused illnesses. He wrote:

"[S]urvival rates for the most common types of cancer—those which make up 90 percent of the cases—have remained virtually unchanged over the last twenty-five years. This fact has consistently been clouded by announcements from the American Cancer Society reminiscent of General Westmoreland's proclamations from Vietnam" (191).

In 1978, Prof. Samuel S. Epstein of the University of Illinois published his classic, *The Politics of Cancer*. Although this dealt mainly with the link between environmental pollution and malignancy, its unwavering criticism of the "cancer establishment" laid the basis for much that followed. Dr. Epstein has kept up a concerted campaign since then, often through the op-ed pages of various leading newspapers (115).

Fired from Memorial

In November, 1977, I myself was fired from my position as assistant director of public affairs at MSKCC after I blew the whistle on a cover-up of positive experiments with nontoxic cancer treatments. In 1980 I published *The Cancer Syndrome* (revised and republished in 1989 as *The Cancer Industry*). This dealt mainly with the question of "unproven" treatments, but also contained an analysis of the failures of the "proven therapies," especially chemotherapy. The book was rather widely reviewed, serialized in magazines and newspapers, and discussed on "60 Minutes" (269).

Thomas L. Dao, head of Roswell Park Memorial Institute's Department of Breast Surgery wrote in a collection of essays celebrating that institution's 75th anniversary that "despite improved surgical techniques, advanced methods of radiotherapies, and widespread use of chemotherapies, breast cancer mortality has not changed in the last 70 years" (156).

Scientific American critique

As noted, in November, 1985, Prof. John Cairns published a lead article on the war on cancer in the *Scientific American* (60). Its appearance in that prestigious non-specialized journal marked the beginning of the end of uncritical public support for the war. It became acceptable to cast a cold eye on many of the claims of the cancer establishment.

In May, 1986 came another devastating blow. The former editor of the *Journal of the National Cancer Institute*, John C. Bailar III, M.D., Ph.D., chair of the department of epidemiology and biostatistics of McGill University, Montreal, and his University of Iowa colleague Dr. Elaine M. Smith, published an historic study of overall survival data in the *New England Journal of Medicine* (28). Bailar had previously published a celebrated critique of the NCI's mammography program (27).

A qualified failure

The purpose of Bailar and Smith's "Special Article" was to "assess the overall progress against cancer during the years 1950 to 1982," the last year for which reliable data was available to them.

"It is time for open debate to take stock of past achievements and to consider" what should be invested in future efforts, they added.

While the Cairns critique was basically clinical and biological, the Bailar-Smith article looked at the problem from the point of view of epidemiology and statistics. "We come to similar conclusions about the poor rate of success to date," Bailar and Smith wrote about Cairns, and both articles should be read together "for a more comprehensive view of the matter."

"Some 35 years of intense and growing efforts to improve the treatment of cancer have not had much overall effect on the most fundamental measure of clinical outcome—death," said Bailar and Smith. "Overall," they wrote, "the effort to control cancer has failed—so far—to attain its objectives."

They call this a "generally dismal picture," brightened somewhat by the decreased mortality in those under 30. They also point out that "such deaths account for only about one to two percent of total mortality from cancer" (28).

In a now-famous statement they wrote, "The main conclusion we draw is that some 35 years of intense effort focused largely on improving treatment must be judged a qualified failure. Results have not been what they were intended and expected to be" (28).

Chemo's Berlin Wall

And then, in 1990, came a 92-page monograph, *The Chemotherapy of Advanced Epithelial Cancer* by Dr. Ulrich Abel (3,4). Abel is a biostatistician at the Institute for Epidemiology and Biometry of the University of Heidelberg, Germany. Abel previously studied the effectiveness of cancer drugs from a rigorous and generally sympathetic point of view. Like Cairns, Bailar and Bross, he was well situated to objectively assess the successes and failures of an establishment of which he himself is a member.

Abel's critique focused on the question of whether chemotherapy was indeed effective in prolonging survival in advanced epithelial cancers. His answer was that it had not. Abel raised the stakes by summarizing and extending such findings and coming to an overall conclusion about chemotherapy in general. He also pointed out the lack of good studies demonstrating actual palliation through cytotoxic drugs. Abel courageously asked the most important questions that could be asked about cancer chemotherapy. These questions still demand answers.

Rigorous proof lacking

In *The Cancer Industry*, I attempted to document the failure of the establishment to carry out rigorous examinations of alternative treatments (269). But reading Abel, I realized that rigorous demonstrations of life-prolongation rarely take place before chemotherapy is put into practice.

People in general, Abel remarked, "take it for granted that if a notoriously toxic and expensive treatment cannot cure, it must at least have some beneficial effect on the patient's prognosis." They take it for granted, because they have been subjected to a media barrage about impending successes with new drugs. But they are wrong.

You might think that a book such as Abel's would have triggered a revolution. It did provoke serious discussion in Germany, including a favorable article in the newsweekly, *Der Spiegel*. But in the United States, birthplace of chemotherapy, it was virtually ignored, although the book itself was written in English.

In December, 1990, I wrote a review in the newsletter I edit, *The Cancer Chronicles*, comparing its publication to the then-current destruction of the Berlin Wall. But a recent search turned up no reviews of this work in other American publications. This, I believe, is not because it was unimportant, but on the contrary because its arguments were irrefutable. They were answered by the most effective argument of all—silence.

Braverman's modest proposal

In 1991, Albert S. Braverman, M.D., Professor of Hematology and Oncology of the Health Sciences Center at the State University of New York, Brooklyn gave an insider's view of the war on cancer in *The Lancet*, with the deceptively mild title, "Medical Oncology in the 1990s" (48).

In it, he proposed a logical solution to the chemotherapy problem. "The time has come," he wrote, "to cut back on the clinical investigation of new chemotherapeutic regimens for cancer and to cast a critical eye on the way chemotherapeutic treatment is now being administered."

The name of the game

The reader might wonder how the chemotherapy establishment could ignore such a long string of trenchant criticisms. The answer is complex, but one sociological explanation is given by Dr. Irwin Bross. Bross, a 30-year veteran of the cancer war, is the author of 400 scientific articles; his opinions should therefore carry some weight. According to him, "in an establishment, status is the name of the game"; but in the medical establishment, contrary to public perception, scientists are second-class citizens.

At most institutions (but not including the Roswell Park of his day), medical doctors are paid far more and only their opinions count. Ironically, says Bross, M.D.s who become scientists (rather than clinicians or administrators) are also looked down upon, while "scientists without an M.D. have much the same status as other paramedicals in the health care game" (55). Under such a schema, you can imagine what is thought of criticism from non-scientists, patients, or the general public: they simply fall off the map!

Personal attacks

Unable to adequately answer their critics' arguments, promoters of chemotherapy fall back on the time-honored technique of attacking the qualifications, motives, and personalities of their critics. Personal attacks are common in the defense of chemotherapy and have become a marked feature of the debate. This is quite the opposite of the public's idea of science as an objective and dispassionate calling, unmarred by ugly tactics.

In 1978, French oncologist Lucien Israel ascribed a natural skepticism about intensive chemotherapy to the "paranoia, vanity, [and] careerism" of his opponents. They simply do not subscribe to the right journals, he said, are lazy, out-of-date, or are simply not behaving as adults. Or they are cowards who are afraid of death and need to "become converts to rationality."

When John Bailar criticized some aspects of the war on cancer, Vincent T. DeVita, Jr., M.D., then the NCI director, claimed that Dr. Bailar had "departed with reality." And the president of the American Society of Clinical Oncology called this world-famous biostatistician "the great nay sayer of our time" (269).

Similarly, when Martin Shapiro, M.D. of the University of California at Los Angeles criticized in the *Los Angeles Times* what he felt was unnecessary chemotherapy, he was hit with a barrage of criticism.

UCLA oncologist Gregory Sarna claimed that Shapiro, an internist, did not have the "background" to understand the benefits of chemotherapy for pancreatic or lung cancer. It was his lack of "experience" that led him to claim that chemo frequently causes side effects (332).

"I couldn't help but think of the many patients I have treated who have benefited from chemotherapy, who might have not tried such therapy had they read his article," wrote Sarna (332). By giving an honest account of chemotherapy, based on first-hand experiences, Shapiro was practically accused of contributing to the death of cancer patients.

People generally resort to personal attacks when they sense that their arguments are weak or fatally flawed. Chemotherapists cannot help but suspect that their field rests on a bed of sand. They try to distract attention from this fact by launching personal attacks against those who point out the problems.

Ad hominem attacks can be very damaging, however. They can also be the prelude to worse things: a withdrawal of funding and referrals, for instance. In 1966, after Dr. Bross and four colleagues published a series of groundbreaking articles with the title "Is Toxicity Really Necessary?" (51,52,53) they lost their government support for drug testing studies. The NCI doctor in charge, Bross recalled, "had a very satisfied look on his face when he cut off our funding" (55).

CHAPTER THREE
The Profession of Oncology

OVER THE PAST TWENTY YEARS I have heard many stories about how people are treated by their oncologists. Some of these are truly heartening and there are clearly many caring individuals out there. More often, however, I have been shocked by some of the profession's lack of empathy and sensitivity in both language and behavior.

Studies have shown that in the average office visit "physicians actually spend 1.3 minutes or less giving information, but *believed* that they had spent nearly seven times as long on that task." Patients, locked into a passive conception of their role, averaged only *eight seconds* asking questions (228).

In my own experience at MSKCC, the way I heard doctors speaking to and about their patients added to my growing disillusionment with the war on cancer. For instance, I routinely heard some doctors refer to their advanced patients as "waste-basket cases." I heard the widely used drug BCNU jokingly referred to as "Be seein' you," and 5-FU as "Five Feet Under."

At Grand Rounds early one morning, a prominent doctor displayed a *Playboy* centerfold and said, "Some of our patients look like this." He then displayed the picture of a seriously overweight woman, her breasts hanging down to her waist. "Others," he said, "look like this." Another celebrated surgeon whom I interviewed for *Center News* had a lamp in the shape of a woman's breast on his office desk. I was so astonished I could hardly get out a single question.

Have doctors changed? In 1994, the *New York Times* described a top clinical researcher as "self-confident with a manner that is often perceived as arrogant and abrasive" (4/4/94).

Liberal arts clichés

What I hear from people with cancer often supports this impression. When a young woman of my acquaintance expressed reservations about taking aggressive chemotherapy for her stage I ovarian cancer, her oncologist dismissed them as "Liberal Arts clichés" and "over-intellectualizing." A man wrote to the newsletter I edit, *The Cancer Chronicles*, complaining that after his diagnosis with advanced cancer, "Immediate high-dosage chemotherapy was described as my only way to stay alive. I actually had a hard time leaving the clinic. Only after I agreed to start the chemo protocol by the weekend, did the oncologist agree to let me be."

Many patients are not so resourceful, however, and passively accept whatever their oncologist pressures them to do. (A "patient," after all is defined by Webster as "one who is acted upon.")

I hear about doctors who deliver a virtual death sentence on a fellow human being, and then turn on their heels and walk out. The language that some doctors use is shocking. Brown University historian James Patterson tells the story of a surgeon who informed "the family of a man on whom he had just operated that the patient was 'rotten clear through'" (295). Cancer doctors routinely say that their patients "failed" the treatment, when in fact they mean that the treatment failed the patient. They also routinely refer to their patients as if they were mere vehicles for their disease.

"I saw five breast cancers in my office today," a doctor once told me.

"Really," I let slip, "Were there any people attached?"

I am sure there is some compensatory mechanism at work here. One oncologist has told how "the patient's and physician's anxiety about the disease and the toxic treatments...hamper reasoned discussions and charge the atmosphere with hidden messages. The physician's own fears of death and failure to cure enhance the intensity of this interchange" (376).

Existential fear

French oncologist Lucien Israel, M.D. has written at length about some cancer doctors' existential fear or even loathing of their own patients, who, he says, represent their own powerlessness against death (193).

One must sympathize with doctors who must endure mind-numbing duty, day in and day out. Yet, all the same, the stories one hears are shocking, and are rarely ever given public exposure. One muted, but devastating, criticism appeared in an article in the *New York Times Magazine* (12/4/94). Novelist Robert Kotlowitz told the story of his own wife's death from lung cancer.

Their unnamed doctor, Kotlowitz reported, started almost every sentence with the word 'unfortunately'—a "compulsive verbal tic," Kotlowitz calls it. The doctor scheduled Mrs. Kotlowitz to have chemotherapy just three days after her life-shattering diagnosis. Here is a sample of their colloquy:

" 'And suppose I decide not to have chemotherapy,' she asked. 'What would my life expectancy be?'

" 'Perhaps six to eight months,' the doctor said, hesitating only a moment. 'Are you considering such a choice?'
" 'No,' my wife said, getting up to leave. 'Just curiosity.'
" 'Good,' the doctor said. 'Because treatment is important.' "

Later, viewing his wife when she was dying, Kotlowitz wrote with his novelist's eye:

"I begin to think of the photographs I have seen of the first debilitated casualties of poison gas during World War I....My wife suffers from the same helplessness, the same enfeeblement after chemotherapy, with one major difference: she suffers under medical guidance."

Deception

Deception has a long, albeit rarely told, history in the cancer field. Not long ago, it was standard practice not to tell patients they even had a life-threatening illness, or to mention the word "cancer" in their presence. It is worth looking at what was standard practice just a generation ago.

In a 1955 book, *Should the Patient Know the Truth?*, two dozen experts (doctors, nurses, ministers, etc.) were asked if patients, and particularly cancer patients, should even be told the truth about their condition (353). Only a handful answered at all positively. Instead, the book is scattered throughout with astonishing sentiments, all on the theme that "most cancer patients do not want to know the truth."

A psychiatrist at New York's Mt. Sinai Hospital actually said that doctors are "endowed with attributes of omnipotence and omniscience," but should "use that power with wisdom and restraint...." Or as the old joke has it, "That's God—he thinks he's a doctor!"

A nursing executive dutifully reports, "When a patient says to the nurse, 'Do I have cancer?' the nurse simply asks, 'Do you think you have cancer?' Usually the conversation changes to something else and no more mention is made of cancer" (353). End of story.

Will-o'-the-wisp

The co-editor of *Should the Patient Know the Truth?* counsels doctors to tell their cancer patients that "experimental drugs are being used now," when in fact he had to know that few drugs were then available, and none had relevance to the overwhelming majority of the cancers being treated by his readers.

So why the deception? So that patients, he says, will not "begin hunting about for that will-o'-the-wisp, a cancer cure...." In other words, doctors should give patients highly toxic but ineffective drugs just to keep them out of the hands of "a charlatan who promises results while he impoverishes the family" (354.) This is echoed in a 1970s textbook from the ACS, in which chemotherapy is promoted as a way of "preventing improper orientation of the patient" (321).

Only one of the doctors in the 1955 book responded with an unambiguous defense of truth-telling:

"The most important person in an illness is the patient himself," Owen H. Wangensteen, M.D., Ph.D. of the University of Minnesota wrote. "Yet, physicians frequently follow a policy of dissimulation in acquainting patients with the nature of a cancerous malady." Such lies, white or otherwise, violate "that sincerity and truth which the patient rightfully may expect of his physician" (388).

Wangensteen accused doctors and family members of spinning a web of "conspiracy" around the patient, which made the patient mistrust his physician and the "insincere behavior of his family."

Deceptively rosy picture

In conclusion, he warned his fellow doctors:

"We are all being examined every day, perhaps not by judges of the law but by persons whose clarity and acuity of vision in this important matter transcends our own" (388).

What a wonderful statement—and what a contrast to the majority sentiment at that time.

Even in the late 1960s, according to veteran science writer Victor Cohen of the *Washington Post*, "doctors either didn't tell patients 'it's cancer' or painted a deceptively rosy picture between 70 and 90 percent of the time" (78).

Although this sort of deception about the diagnosis is still said to be common in Japan, it is now far less common in America and most of Western Europe. Since the late 1970s, said Cohen, more than 90 percent of Western physicians "always" or "usually" make full disclosure. Today, the main arena of deception has shifted to the realm of prognosis, i.e., the likely outcome, of advanced or metastatic cancer, as well as the likely effects and side effects of chemotherapy.

Patients with advanced disease are often told that their treatment will do more good than it is likely to do. This deception can take many forms, but usually central to the act is the presentation of chemotherapy as more effective (and less toxic) than it really is.

For example, a woman wrote to the *Los Angeles Times* about her father who was receiving aggressive chemotherapy for his pancreatic cancer.

"Unable to ignore my increasingly gaunt and yellowing father, I asked the doctor, privately, what really was going on. Exuberantly he supplied the analogy of my father as being a car in perfect working condition except for an old tire. 'Now, that tire may never be "same" again, but otherwise, that car will last forever!' I believe he pounded his fist somewhere during the last few words.

"Two days later, age 51, Dad died, the cancer having spread throughout his body. "Inexplicable!" she exclaims, ironically (365).

Understating side effects

Doctors also routinely understate the likely side effects of chemotherapy. They find allies among a minority of patients who attest to little or no negative reactions to these drugs. Such a downplaying of chemotherapy's toxicity can backfire, however. For example, when advice columnist Ann Landers printed a letter from a woman who described her own post-mastectomy chemotherapy as a "breeze," this was too much for many readers.

From Vancouver, a woman wrote:

"The doctor ordered chemo, the whole load. I was exhausted and depressed, sick as a dog, and I couldn't keep food down."

A woman in San Diego wrote that while her own treatment was mild "sometimes treatment can go on for a year or more, resulting in total hair loss, vomiting and loss of appetite." Another woman in Minnesota, whose husband was successfully treated for Hodgkin's disease, wrote that, nonetheless, he "went through hell. The side effects were a nightmare" (224).

A Japanese view

It is often said that the Japanese trail Americans in regard to medical candor (216). But when a Japanese doctor, Naoko T. Miyaji, M.D., looked at this question he was shocked to learn that even in the 1990s, American physicians were not as candid with advanced patients as they claimed to be (262,263).

For instance, he found that they routinely withheld crucial information on the grounds that patients are unwilling to know the truth. They often stated that the individual's future is uncertain or irrelevant to immediate medical action.

They also cited the need to preserve the patient's hope, although the treatments they proposed in fact offered little or no realistic basis for optimism.

In a letter to the *New England Journal of Medicine*, Dr. Miyaji explained that withholding the prognosis (which often includes

QUESTIONING CHEMOTHERAPY

misrepresenting the effectiveness of chemotherapy) can "harm the patient-doctor relationship" and—in bold words for an M.D.—"serve the interests of oncologists and pharmaceutical companies at the sacrifice of patients' time, money, and quality of life" (263).

Hypocrisy
It is also relevant to ask what oncologists themselves do when they get cancer. Do they believe in their own treatments so much that they take it themselves and recommend it for their family members? I had reason to doubt it. I remembered the story of a celebrated Sloan-Kettering chemotherapist who, when he found out that he had advanced cancer, told his colleagues, "Do anything you want—but no chemotherapy!" It was an open secret that an official of Sloan-Kettering Institute sent his mother to Germany for unconventional treatment.

Yet, there have been only a few studies that attempt to answer such a potentially illuminating question. The most rigorous of them was carried out in Canada—and its implications are devastating.

In 1986, McGill Cancer Center scientists sent a questionnaire to 118 doctors who treated non-small-cell lung cancer (NSCLC). All of them were affiliated with the Princess Margaret Hospital in Toronto or with the Ontario Cancer Research and Treatment Foundation, which operates seven cancer clinics throughout the province (243). More than three-quarters of them recruited patients and then helped carry out clinical trials of new drugs for lung cancer.

These Canadian specialists were asked to imagine that they themselves had non-small-cell lung cancer. NSCLC is a cancer that is commonly treated with toxic drugs. In fact, according to an orthodox textbook, "All appropriate patients with inoperable NSCLC should be encouraged to participate in clinical trials as initial therapy" (141).

The doctors were asked which of six different randomized chemotherapy trials they would choose to enter.

Specialists would not consent
When it came to themselves, "most specialists who treat lung cancer would not consent to participate as subjects in many of these trials," according to the Canadian survey. Sixty-four out of 79 respondents (81 percent) said they would not consent to be in a drug trial that contained cisplatin, a drug noted for its extreme toxicity.

And of these 64, 58 found *all* the drug trials unacceptable. Their main reasons? The ineffectiveness of chemotherapy and its unacceptable degree of toxicity.

40

"[Chemotherapy] was uniformly unpopular regardless of the background and experience of the subjects," the Canadian report noted dryly.

The more familiar these doctors were with a particular treatment, in fact, the less likely they were to accept it for themselves. "Fifty-four percent of those who treated more than 50 new lung cancer patients each year rejected all or all but one of the six studies, compared to 35 percent of those who treated fewer new cases.

In an accompanying editorial in the *Journal of Clinical Oncology*, Dr. Heine H. Hansen of the Finsen Institute, Copenhagen, who carried out such trials, concurred: "Based on the existing literature, it is difficult not to concur with our colleagues" in not taking treatments, he wrote. He added, "One can question the justification of continuing therapeutic trials along these lines in non-small-cell lung cancer" (166).

Abel makes an inquiry

In March, 1989, German biostatistician Dr. Ulrich Abel undertook his own systematic investigation of physicians' own choices in cancer treatment. He received 150 replies to a letter of inquiry sent to oncologists and research units around the world, trying to gauge these doctors' feelings about the use of chemotherapy in advanced carcinoma.

Essentially, he reported, "the personal views of many oncologists seem to be in striking contrast to communications intended for the public." His findings were in accord with a number of other informal polls that have also shown that many oncologists would decline chemotherapy for themselves or their own families (17,268).

A definition to ponder

Yet the same doctors continue to send patients to oncologists or to prescribe chemotherapy for their own patients. What should we call this? Of course, oncologists are skilled and well-trained professionals, not unscrupulous charlatans. Nevertheless, they might ponder the words of one of their own leaders, Dr. James Holland. In a diatribe against non-conventional doctors, he wrote:

"My definition of cancer quackery is the deliberate misapplication of a diagnostic or treatment procedure in a patient with cancer....[T]he culprit who victimizes his fellow man suffering from cancer, impeding the patient's access to available therapies or constructive investigation, all the while greedily enriching himself, is a quack, a criminal, a jackal among men who deserves the scorn and ostracism of society. Because human life is at stake, he must be controlled" (cited in 225).

When experts refuse to participate

The authors of the Canadian study asked, rhetorically, "If experts refuse to participate in a trial, should uncomprehending patients be asked to consent?" Whether they should or should not is a moot point. It is exactly these doctors, after all, who recruit lung cancer patients to participate in chemotherapy trials.

I am not trying to say that oncologists are bad people. I still believe that many go into that profession because of a sincere desire to help humanity and a hatred for what cancer does to human lives. However, the tools oncologists are working with are barely effective, and are in fact inappropriate to most cancers. The whole military philosophy behind their efforts seems misguided.

At the same time, they are not the beleagured minority they once were. Astonishing profits and worldly success have made some leaders of the field arrogant, at the same time that a gnawing realization of ultimate failure has paradoxically rendered them insecure and defensive.

This is a group that collectively needs to take a long, hard look in the mirror. But human nature being what it is, as long as the money continues to roll in, that is unlikely to happen. It will be the mass defection of patients and changes in government policy that in the end will force necessary changes in the profession of oncology.

CHAPTER FOUR

The Randomized Clinical Trial

TO UNDERSTAND THE CLAIMS MADE for chemotherapy one must understand something about randomized clinical (or controlled) trials (RCTs). The RCT is the main technique used to find out whether or not a drug really works. It is a human experiment in which the effects of one drug (or multi-drug regimen) are directly compared to those of another regimen given to patients with the same diagnosis.

The RCT was invented in an attempt to eliminate the possibility of "serious bias" (35) in studies of new drugs. The need for RCTs stems from the fact that many people make claims for treatments that are subject to error, misinterpretation, or even fraud.

Patient Testimonials

Throughout most of history, "proof" of the safety and effectiveness of a new drug was provided by testimonials from satisfied patients or their doctors, which were then publicized by the drug's manufacturer. Many people now feel that such testimonials smack of charlatanism. But until the end of World War II, few saw any major problems with this system. However, it was seriously flawed.

Patients and doctors often have all sorts of ideas about what is helping them. For example, millions of people have been diagnosed with cancer, yet are still alive. Some believe they were saved by surgery or radiation. Others credit diet, herbs, or a deep, abiding faith in God. Still others are convinced that chemotherapy was instrumental in saving or prolonging their lives.

"If it were not for surgery and aggressive chemotherapy, I would not be here to write this letter," a woman with colon cancer wrote the *Los Angeles Times*. But how does this woman know that chemotherapy led to her long-term survival? After all, the majority of people with colon cancer, even those with regionally spread disease, survive five years with surgery alone.

Another woman claimed that "after only two chemotherapy treatments, there is no x-ray evidence of one tumor....Thanks to chemotherapy I am presently in remission....I feel I've been given another lease on life" (185). The remission has given her hope. But is this realistic or "false hope"—exactly what the chemotherapists accuse alternative doctors of purveying?

A UCLA oncologist related the heartening story of a young man with colon cancer who recovered and then went on to father two children. I have heard scores of such anecdotes from oncologists. How does one answer these individuals?

Compelling personal stories

Well, personal stories are compelling, but are usually inconclusive. Sometimes people get the facts wrong, even about their own cases. Others attribute benefit to one part of the treatment (e.g., chemotherapy) when the real benefit came from another part (e.g., surgery). At other times, the person unfortunately speaks too soon, and will not actually survive longer than the average untreated patient. Cancers can even reoccur after many years, after the person has been officially entered into the "cure" statistics.

People also hesitate to criticize treatments into which they have invested a great deal of time, money, and effort. There is an almost superstitious dread of saying anything bad about a treatment that you feel is keeping you alive. The walls have ears.

I do not wish to denigrate another individual's experience or choice in taking any treatment. Cancer is far too complicated a problem to allow for any dogmatism. However, it is necessary to carefully examine any such account, and to remain respectfully skeptical of the details.

And even if a "cure" can truly be documented, we must acknowledge that there is almost always some peculiar combination of factors that went into such a success. A friend of mine is often cited as a famous success story of conventional methods. Yet he turns out to have also utilized unconventional immune treatments and intensive guided visualization to aid in his recovery. So was it the chemotherapy? Or was it his intensive efforts at visualizing his cancer melting away? Who can say?

History of randomized clinical trial

It is because of the uncertainties surrounding the analysis of individual cases that scientists have evolved a way of studying the effects of new treatments, the randomized clinical trial (RCT).

Essentially, in the RCT, the patients in question are assigned to an "arm" of the study in what is called a non-deliberate fashion, without choice or bias. To put it in medical jargon, they are "randomized." These patients are then compared not just to "controls" (who do not receive the treatment in question) but to "concurrent controls," since historical comparisons are regarded as unreliable and actually "may confound the treatment comparison" (35).

The RCT was first suggested in the 1930s by the great British statistician, Austin Bradford Hill. The first such test was conducted in Great Britain between 1946 and 1948: a now-famous investigation of the drug streptomycin for tuberculosis, for which Hill provided the statistical analysis (84,379).

While some RCTs were carried out in the 1950s, the main impetus for their proliferation came from the 1962 Kefauver-Harris amendments to the U.S. Food, Drug and Cosmetic Act. This historic law called for "substantial evidence" to prove the effectiveness of any new drug marketed in the United States. This law has greatly influenced practice in many other countries, as well.

Substantial evidence

At the time, the phrase "substantial evidence" was vaguely interpreted to mean "adequate and well-controlled investigations, including clinical investigations." The lawmakers were not necessarily thinking of randomized clinical trials when they wrote this language. "The phrase was used as the scientific analog of the legal phrase 'substantial evidence,' (i.e., more than an iota, less than a preponderance)" (373). However, before long, the FDA interpreted that requirement to mean at least two randomized studies.

This launched a whole new research establishment that provided RCTs to a burgeoning medical-industrial complex, and incidentally gave work to thousands of people. Eventually, an entangled financial web of government, academia, and industry developed. Drug makers established networks of principal investigators at some of the leading research and treatment centers in the United States and abroad.

Need for RCTs

With treatments that are dramatically effective there is no need for RCTs. Thus, there has never been a trial of aspirin for headache. Nor was there a controlled clinical trial of penicillin for bacterial infection nor of insulin for diabetes (37). However, even in such cases RCTs might still be desirable, since doctors are sometimes mistaken as a group about the effectiveness of a favorite treatment (305).

"The essence of a clinical trial is comparison," according to two British statisticians writing in the excellent review of such trials, *Randomized Trials in Cancer: A Critical Review by Sites*, prepared for the European Organization for Research and Treatment of Cancer (EORTC) (346). In its essence, the RCT compares treatments using a sample of present-day patients in order to identify how best to treat future patients. The emphasis is on the future: not everyone in the

RCT can possibly receive optimal treatment.

In cancer, RCTs began to be used on a large scale in the 1950s. They soon became a part of medical-social belief and were seen as the "only scientifically respectable method for comparing treatments" (35). Their growth paralleled that of the chemotherapy enterprise. When trials at one institution were found to be insufficient to yield answers, whole networks of medical centers were strung together into clinical trial groups, most of them testing complex combinations of agents.

As of 1995, there were almost 300,000 articles referring to cytotoxic agents listed in the National Library of Medicine's "MEDLARS" database. Among these were the results of thousands of clinical trials. In one year alone, 1990, the National Cancer Institute was sponsoring ten major cooperative clinical trial groups, involving more than 4,600 clinical investigators conducting approximately 400 protocol studies on more than 23,000 patients with cancer. The cost of these trials in one year was over $60 million (135).

Direct evidence

There are three kinds of studies that can provide direct evidence of a new drug's effectiveness.

Randomized comparisons of patients treated with a drug vs. patients not treated with the drug

In such studies, the patients must be assigned in advance to what are called the arms of the study in a non-deliberate, non-purposeful manner, using a truly random or non-decipherable mechanism (97). The "controls" in such an experiment are individuals with cancer who receive either no treatment or get a placebo—an inert and therapeutically worthless substance. In either case, they do not receive the drug or drugs under study. This is the classic "placebo-controlled study," which many regard as the gold standard of tests.

If the drug under review is compared to an inert substance (a saline injection, for example, or a sugar pill), then it is called a placebo-controlled study. And when neither doctor nor patient knows who gets what, this is called a double-blind study.

Many people, even doctors, naively identify RCTs with "double-blind, placebo-controlled" trials. The two are not synonymous, and in fact it is not always necessary or possible to make trials double-blind. For example, all conventional cancer drugs, as Dr. DeVita has reminded us, have "significant side effects" when used in pharmacological doses (97). And oftentimes, those effects are unique. A comparison of such a drug with an inert placebo must often be based on a polite fiction, since after the very first attack of nausea, or worse, both doctor and patient will know who is getting the toxic agent.

If you are in a "double-blind" study and your urine turns blue, the chances are you are receiving mitoxantrone, not a sugar pill; if it turns bright red, the chances are it's daunorubicin, not a saline injection. Guinea pigs don't read the *PDR* (*Physician's Desk Reference*); human patients have been known to do so.

Such tests are undertaken so that predictions can be made about what generally happens when a new treatment is applied to similar patients, without the interference of confounding subjective factors.

In fact, true placebo controls have been almost abandoned in the testing of chemotherapy. Drug regimen is now generally tested against drug regimen, and doctors hardly look at whether the drugs do better than simple good nursing care. The value of chemotherapy is a given.

Cairns drew our attention to a similar situation in the nineteenth century. At that time, bleeding was the standard therapy for pneumonia. Doctors performed comparative studies to determine the outcome of bleeding at different stages of the disease but no one (at least in the orthodox medical community) "suggested that these patients might actually have done better if they had been left alone." The analogy with chemotherapy is obvious. With cancer, as with pneumonia, "there may be no way of determining whether any particular patient's survival was predestined or should be attributed to the treatment"(60).

Randomized comparison of immediate vs. deferred chemotherapy

In such studies, doctors attempt to show whether or not it makes a difference if chemotherapy is given at once, or if the doctors adopt a wait-and-see attitude, only administering it if the patient's symptoms worsen. Such studies, as we shall see, have had some surprising results.

Dose-effect studies

These tests attempt to find out whether higher doses of drugs cause longer survival. Such studies must be analyzed with great caution in order to avoid misinterpretations. Conclusions about dose-effect relationships that are drawn from the comparison of different studies are not definitive.

For example, if patients in a high-dose study live longer than low-dose ones, one might assume the high-dose regimen is the better of the two. But this is not always true. For often the high-dose study requires that patients be in better overall physical condition before enrolling (so that they can withstand the arduous level of treatment). But this means that patients in the two studies are no longer comparable.

Also, sometimes the higher dose is achieved not by giving more of the drug at each session but by extending the time during which it is administered (the duration of application). Then, by definition, there cannot be any early deaths among the patients who received the high dose of the drug. The analysis of survival then automatically favors the more aggressive treatment (315).

In other studies (25), patients who drop out of the high-dose group because they cannot stand the side effects are excluded from the final analysis.

The result of such a maneuver is also to make the performance of the drug or regimen look better. That is because patients who remain for evaluation are the relatively robust ones. The toxicity of the high-dose group is thereby underestimated and early deaths (whether caused by the disease or by the treatment itself) are either under-represented or are entirely missing from the high-dose group.

All this leads to what are called "artificial dose-effect relationships," and the fostering of grave illusions. In some cases, in fact, the apparent survival advantage of the higher-dose group in reality reflects the harm that is caused by long-term chemotherapy. With good reason, Ulrich Abel calls this situation "particularly disturbing" (3).

Indirect evidence

There are also some forms of evidence that, while only offering indirect proof, do provide useful clues as to whether a drug is effective. Let us consider three kinds of indirect evidence.

Randomized comparisons of two chemotherapy regimens

Patients can be put into two arms, each of which receives a different combination of drugs. This is attractive to many doctors and patients, since at least all participants get a real treatment, not a placebo. But in doing this, the ultimate question of chemotherapy's effectiveness is neatly bypassed. It is the unchallenged assumption that chemotherapy is effective. This has been repeated so often, in so many different ways, that it has now often become "unethical" to withhold chemotherapy!

If one group of drugs proves much better than another, one might logically conclude that it will also be beneficial for patients. As odd as it seems, this is not necessarily true. First of all, one must rule out the possibility that the difference between the two treatments is the result of the more toxic treatment itself killing patients off sooner. Ironically, this sort of result can be misinterpreted to justify the even more extensive use of chemotherapy.

Non-randomized comparisons of patient groups

Basically, "non-randomized" means that proper precautions have simply not been taken in assigning patients to the various arms of the study. Because of this, all sorts of subjective criteria and biases can creep in. For example, sometimes there are big unnoticed differences between groups based on their racial or socioeconomic status. These are a lower grade of studies, and all such informal or ill-designed studies must be treated with great caution. Yet, often "proof" of the effectiveness of chemotherapy turns out to be based on such studies.

Historical trends

Finally, there is the data derived from historical trends, such as those published by the Surveillance, Epidemiology, and End Results (SEER) Program of the National Cancer Institute. These are cancer incidence and mortality statistics derived from only five states: Connecticut, Hawaii, Iowa, New Mexico, and Utah, as well as four metropolitan areas: Detroit, Atlanta, San Francisco-Oakland, and Seattle-Puget Sound (323).

Such historical trends have been proposed as evidence for the effectiveness of the aggressive treatment for cancer. Whenever there is any upward tick in the survival curve, this is presented as proof of chemotherapy's effectiveness and as the basis for increased government funding for cancer research.

But national death rates vary for reasons other than treatment. For example, we can see that deaths from lung cancer are way up (presumably due to cigarette smoking). Conversely, deaths from cervical cancer are down (presumably due to the Pap smear test and better hygiene). Sometimes rates go down for no apparent reason, as has been the case with stomach cancer in the U.S., which has been declining steadily throughout the twentieth century.

Dr. Elaine M. Rankin, of Guy's Hospital, London, has made the important point that "there has been an improvement in survival even of untreated patients [with NSCLC, ed.] over the years." That is why comparisons with historical controls can be misleading or invalid (314).

Significant effects of better treatments can sometimes be reflected in the national statistics on cancer mortality, but the change has to be dramatic to do so.

In the period 1986 to 1987, for example, the death rate from acute lymphocytic leukemia was about half of what it was in the period 1973 to 1974. For most of the other malignant diseases of children, the percentage changes were equally dramatic. There is little doubt that this was the result of improved treatment.

But aside from the above-mentioned rare cancers, says John Cairns, "it is not possible to detect any sudden changes in the death rates for any of the major cancers that could be credited to chemotherapy" (60).

Overall, the figures for cancer are not encouraging and do not support the idea that modern treatments have made much of a difference. They show that between 1975 and 1991, the age-adjusted cancer mortality rates increased from 162.3 per 100,000 population to 173.4 per 100,000. Thus, there are more cancer deaths, not less.

Even if one excludes cancers of the lung and bronchus (the fastest growing component), one finds that the figure in 1975 was 125.3 and in 1991 it was 123.2 per 100,000, a decline of 0.1 percent (323).

Improvements in supportive care

Unfavorable statistics in cancer are often either ignored or ascribed to that useful bugaboo, smoking. The fact is, however, that not all the increases in cancer incidence and mortality can be laid at the door of tobacco. There are a number of technical reasons why survival rates may increase, other than improved therapy.

For example, there is the important question of what effect early detection has on the statistics. (We shall deal with this in some depth in the section on lead-time bias.)

There has also been an intensification and general improvement in the supportive care of patients. In olden days, advanced patients were treated very poorly, and presumably died more quickly. In 1974, America's first hospice opened in New Haven, Connecticut. By 1990, there were almost 2,000 American hospices and 200 Canadian facilities (49). Presumably, this one change alone should have made a difference in survival statistics between 1974 and twenty years later.

Improvement may also be attributable to more sanitary operating rooms, or improved nursing care. Thus, in all likelihood, patients are surviving longer today than they did decades ago. But it is totally unwarranted to lay this laudable progress at the feet of chemotherapy. There are also changes in the structure of various patient groups as well as differences in both the quality of disease monitoring and in data collection.

In many kinds of cancer there has been a standoff in cancer survival rates. In a classic New Haven study by Yale professor Alvan Feinstein, a reason for this standoff is suggested. According to Prof. Feinstein, the benefits of better supportive care for some patients are being wiped out by the "detrimental complications in others" receiving chemotherapy. "The opposing effects," Feinstein says, "in different patients have counterbalanced one another statistically" (119). The results in chemotherapy have apparently dragged down the better results in patients receiving just good supportive care.

SEER data

It is common to argue from historical data, however, that great progress is being made. In the summer of 1994, there was a report from the Canadian province of British Columbia claiming that "survival among women with breast cancer improved significantly…during the period when adjuvant systemic therapy became widely used" (289).

In early 1995, new data from the SEER program was used to further promote "adjuvant" chemotherapy among women with breast cancer.

In his farewell address to the National Cancer Advisory Board, NCI director Dr. Samuel Broder said that there was a "clear decline" in deaths due to breast cancer in American women of 4.7 percent from 1989 to 1992. The decline for white women was 5.5 percent. Among black women, however, the rate went up 2.6 percent.

"This is the largest short-term decline in the breast cancer death rate since 1950," he said. "For white women, the decline is seen in virtually every age group." Almost all white women show some evidence of a downturn in slope after 1990, from 3.4 to 9.3 percent.

He pointed out that from 1987 to 1992 there had been a roughly 18 percent decline in the death rate for white women aged 30 to 39.

Broder admits that "much research will be necessary to understand the specific reasons for the decline," but attributed some of the decline to adjuvant therapy for breast cancer (after potentially curative surgery). However, his boss, HHS Secretary Donna E. Shalala, was far more cautious in her interpretation, stating "We do not know if this trend will hold for the long term, we do not have a thorough understanding of the causes, and we are still very far from seeing a positive trend for all American women. The job before us remains immense" (375). Most scholars hesitated to make definitive statements based on such statistics.

Unwarranted assumptions

Those with the greatest stake in the war on cancer jumped forward with unwarranted assumptions. "This is very encouraging news," said Dr. Robert A. Smith of the American Cancer Society. "We invested in research and it looks like it has paid off. And with some other drugs coming on line, and screening continuing to increase, it is possible that the trend will continue" (179).

The implication is clearly that chemotherapy is doing its job —the more the better. One certainly cannot rule out the possible contribution of chemotherapy to this decline. However, it is important to remember that the actual reasons for this decline (as for many of the ups and downs in cancer statistics) are not known. Statisticians tell us that unless the results are very dramatic, this sort of historical analysis is regarded by statisticians as the weakest form of indirect evidence.

In the words of M.K. Palmer of the Holt Radium Institute in Manchester, "Mortality statistics are of limited value in survival studies of cancer patients" (293).

A 1993 monograph of the NCI itself, written when the downturn in breast cancer mortality was already under way, remarked that "recent breast cancer mortality patterns in young women have been studied and found to be most likely associated with a cohort effect rather than with an effect of treatment" (260). This means that it is probably something about the life style of the women themselves rather than medical intervention that is responsible for the declining death rate.

The way to solve these questions is by carrying out adequate randomized clinical trials. As we shall see, however, really definitive studies are rarely carried out, and when they are, they often prove embarrassing to advocates of cytotoxic chemotherapy.

CHAPTER FIVE

The Problem of Fraud

⌒

"Many excellent notions or experiments are,
by sober and modest men, suppressed."
—Robert Boyle, 1661 (162)

BEFORE WE CONSIDER THE RESULTS that have been achieved with randomized clinical trials (RCTs) in cancer, we must first deal with another problem in interpreting clinical trials. This is the existence of widespread bias and even fraud in the conduct of such trials. The record of oncologists in this regard has not been spotless.

Throughout 1994, headlines were filled with stories of fraud uncovered within one of the largest and most important chemotherapy testing programs in the world, the National Surgical Adjuvant Breast and Bowel Project (NSABP) (12). Chemotherapists at a number of medical centers participating in this project, most prominently the St. Luc Hospital in Montreal, Canada, enrolled inappropriate patients in these studies, a practice that could easily have skewed the results in the direction desired by rogue researchers.

This was no minor problem. St. Luc alone contributed 10.5 percent of all patients to at least one study (the so-called B-13). This project had reported "disease-free survival" in women with breast cancer who received adjuvant chemotherapy. A re-analysis of the St. Luc data reported that the "suggestions of benefit" for patients receiving chemotherapy for breast cancer was in fact "diminished" (275,276). To illustrate, according to the NCI re-analysis, at five years, 81.6 percent of control patients survived vs. 86.4 percent of those receiving chemotherapy. When the St. Luc data was excluded, the difference after five years between the two curves narrowed from 4.7 to 4.1 percent. Thus, the study lost some of its already minor significance.

Earthquake

This episode, and the in-fighting that followed, struck like an earthquake in the cancer establishment (12). There was consternation when it turned out that problems had in fact been detected three years earlier by the federal Office of Research Integrity, but no one told the NCI, the *New England Journal of Medicine* (which published a key study), or participants in the study, until an exposé broke in the *Chicago Tribune*.

In the midst of the St. Luc scandal, the NCI discovered that "the NSABP had failed to inform it of another apparent data falsification in a different breast cancer study at a second Montreal hospital," according to the *Tribune* (86). "Further investigation by federal officials and a University of Pittsburgh panel turned up additional instances of questionable data from 11 other NSABP sites," according to the *Washington Post* (3/8/95), "and criticized [Dr. Bernard] Fisher and his staff for dealing carelessly with such cases."

As a result, University of Pittsburgh's Dr. Fisher, one of the leading cancer researchers in the country, was removed from his position as head of the NSABP for "serious management and scientific deficiencies." He was chastised by the NCI director and by members of Congress for having waited eight months before notifying NCI of discrepancies in the Montreal data, and then resisting attempts to improve his auditing procedures and to set up a data safety monitoring board.

In addition, the study continued to collect information on more than three dozen women who had refused to give consent, while properly executed consent forms could not be located for hundreds of other patients (86).

Fisher's response was not reassuring to those concerned about the integrity of clinical trials in general. His answer: "I challenge those in authority to audit other clinical trial databases and see how well they fare" (86).

Recruitment halted

In 1994, the recruitment of patients in many clinical trials was temporarily halted. The resignation of the director of the NCI in late 1994 has also been attributed to fallout from the scandal—the result of his firing Dr. Fisher (249). But despite Fisher's eight-million-dollar lawsuit to regain control of the program, the "future of the NSABP itself is in doubt" (86). In 1995, Fisher also resisted NCI's demand that he swiftly publish a reanalysis of data from one of the disputed studies (250).

The adjuvant treatment of breast cancer with cytotoxic drugs is one of the lynch pins of chemotherapy, and the NSABP was the key element within that program for almost forty years. If this program is seriously marred by cheating and irregularities, what sort of confidence are we supposed to have in the whole U.S. chemo-testing enterprise?

For many people, the main point was forcefully made by Buffalo biostatistician Irwin D. Bross, Ph.D. In a letter to the *New England Journal of Medicine*, he wrote, "...the statistical quality control was grossly inadequate in the NSABP studies. Hence, whether or not some fraudulent cases are eliminated *post hoc*, any findings lack scientific validity" (56).

It will come as a shock to some that fraud and misconduct are not rare events, but are widespread in science. Recent studies have shown that such incidents are not that unusual. For example, a report by the well-respected Acadia Institute showed that 50 percent of faculty members reported that they had been exposed to two or more types of misconduct and questionable research practices (*American Scientist*, 11-12/93).

There is an important economic dimension to this problem, as well, which creates a motive for fraud. Top leaders of the cancer field are themselves often executives, directors, investors, and beneficiaries of the very methods they are supposed to dispassionately investigate. In some cases, whole institutions have sold their intellectual product to drug companies in exchange for vast sums of money, unimaginable just a few decades ago.

Unintentional bias

Not all the errors are the result of conscious cheating, however. A bigger problem may be the very one that clinical trials were designed to overcome—unconscious, unintentional bias. "The whole panoply of statistical tests, estimates, and procedures contains nuances seemingly tailor-made (or perhaps mathematician-made) to confuse the unwary," wrote Temple University mathematician John Allen Paulos in *Discover* magazine (297).

In order to make their results appear better than they really are some researchers employ "strategies of torturing [their] data until it confesses" (348).

"The results of a trial are potentially complicated by bias from a number of sources," wrote Alan J. Wilson and colleagues from the Department of Surgery, King's School of Medicine and Dentistry, London, in the EORTC review (394). "Considerable bias may arise in the selection of patients," says Dr. Elaine M. Rankin (314). She discusses some of the common problems discovered in many papers: inadequate selection of patients; an insufficient number of patients to permit appropriate statistics; the lack of cooperative studies; sloppy adherence to the protocol; the failure to provide a clear statement of "how much of the desired drug dose was actually given over what period of time"; and "how many patients' treatment was reduced or escalated according to predetermined criteria..." (314).

What is surprising is that all of these problems and biases have been fully warned against by eminent clinical statisticians, and many of their instructional articles have been published in leading medical journals and reviews for years. Yet some oncologists continue to make the same mistakes over and over again—as if these pitfalls did not exist and had never been explained to them.

Such obtuseness might be inexplicable, except that it is very much in the interest of some scientists to continue making such "mistakes." Cynics might say that the success of the chemotherapy enterprise actually depends on the perpetuation of errors of this kind.

Responses vs. cures

It is one of the central fallacies of chemotherapy that shrinkages or "response rates" have been proven to correlate with increased survival time. Yet, in answer to a patient's inevitable question, 'What are my chances?' the doctor may give impressive-sounding "response rates" of, say, 60 percent. There is no explanation of what exactly a "response" or a "success" rate is in this context, or how it supposedly correlates with actual increased survival. In fact, such a correlation has not been proven for most kinds of cancer.

Yet time and again, we hear such statements as this:

"We are on the verge of achieving high enough response rates on a consistent basis to affect positively the survival outcome of patients with metastatic non-small-cell lung cancer as a group" (182). Countless other such statements could be given, as this assumption has been repeated so many times that it has taken on the aura of a dogma.

Is it any wonder that many doctors who deal with patients are themselves confused on this point? Or do they know, but are trying to spare a "terminal" patient's feelings? Or are they promoting their services?

The doctor talks "response rate" but the patient hears "cure"! These same patients and their family members may be furious when they realize that "response rates" do not often correlate with increased survival or improved quality of life.

They begin to wonder what in the world is going on—why would doctors lie like this?

The reasoning that connects tumor shrinkages with increased survival is "so obvious and logical that its popularity is hardly surprising," says Dr. Ulrich Abel (3). Yet despite the fact that this is almost universally believed, it happens to be wrong. This is well known to some chemotherapists. According to the outstanding European (EORTC) monograph on breast cancer:

"Response rate alone is a poor parameter by which to assess therapeutic benefit in advanced breast cancer; it does not predict survival, and its effect on quality of life is very much determined by the nature of the treatment used" (241).

Responses vs. survival

The same can be said about many other kinds of cancer. "Response rates" simply do not predict survival in advanced carcinoma, or at least such a theory has never been rigorously proven for the majority of cancer types. This can also be seen quite clearly from the data that a top NCI scientist included in a 1988 contribution to an orthodox text-book of medicine:

Response vs. Disease-Free Survival*

Type of Cancer	Responses	Disease-free survival
Breast, Stages III-IV	75	rare
Small-Cell Lung Cancer	90	10
Stomach	50	rare
Ovarian	75	10-20
Multiple myeloma	75	rare
Acute nonlymphocytic leukemia	75	20
Chronic lymphocytic leukemia	75	rare
Prostate	75	rare
Head and neck	75	rare
Mycosis fungoides	75	rare
Bladder	60	rare

*Data adapted from *Cecil Textbook of Medicine*, 18th Ed., 1988

Yet at scientific meetings (such as those of the American Society for Clinical Oncology) the majority of the abstracts list precisely such "response rates" as the *only* valid criterion for the effectiveness of a new therapy.

To their patients, chemotherapists sometimes speak of the effectiveness of drugs in terms of these "success" or "response rates." Application of drugs may indeed result in a temporary shrinkage of measurable tumors for some patients. But what are the long-term effects of such shrinkages? And to what extent does a "response" really correlate with, or predict, increased survival for the patient? This crucial question is almost never asked—much less answered.

Patient resistance

The scientific argument for RCTs is compelling. How else can one know with any degree of assurance what happens to people when they take a new treatment? How can you find out what is the most effective therapeutic regimen or dose?

It is government policy that all eligible patients should enroll in clinical trials. However, there is a major ethical and logistical dilemma associated with such trials. Most people would not participate in randomized clinical trials, or urge others to, if viable options were available.

As an advanced breast cancer patient said, "It's hard to say, 'I'll be a guinea pig. I want to *live*" (211). One wonders how many of the boosters of clinical trials would actually place themselves, their spouses, parents, or children into such studies. If they really thought there was a potentially curative drug, I suspect they would move heaven and earth to get it for themselves, and stay out of the placebo group.

RCTs in trouble

In fact, a *New York Times* article (9/4/94) stated that nationwide only 3 percent of adults with major illnesses are enrolling in experimental studies that investigate new drugs or therapies to cure disease.

This is generally deplored by the boosters of chemotherapy. Some writers act as if it were one's patriotic duty to join such trials—like voting. But many have figured out that such trials offer a poor deal for medical consumers.

The degree to which patients have deserted such trials was highlighted in another *New York Times* article in 1995. This discussed an NCI study on the treatment of advanced breast cancer.

The study compared an innovative technique that included bone marrow transplantation (BMT) with "the chemotherapy regimes that are now standard treatment." In 18 months, Karen Antman, M.D. of New York's Columbia-Presbyterian "has not enrolled a single woman in the national study." She described herself as "bitterly disappointed." When she tells women that in order for her to treat them they must first enter the study, "they thank her and go elsewhere" (211).

Opposition to RCTs is also running so high among referring physicians that some are now calling her to say, "Don't you dare offer my patient the clinical trial." Doctors are even giving their patients a little chemotherapy before sending them to the hospital, "knowing it makes them ineligible for the trial" (211). RCTs are thus in deep trouble. Patients especially balk at being assigned to arms of the study that consist of either placebo or some already discredited treatment.

Ironically, the main charge that orthodox doctors use against alternative practitioners is that they do not prove their methods by RCTs. Dr. Gregory A. Curt has said that both orthodox and alternative methods should "be evaluated and prioritized" using the same criteria and that "unorthodox approaches should play on a level field with orthodox medicine" (87). Curt and many of his colleagues routinely denigrate alternative therapies for allegedly relying on informal "anecdotal" reports of success rather than on controlled trials.

This assumes that conventional doctors themselves demonstrate through controlled trials that their drugs really extend the life of patients. However, this is not generally the case.

"The reproach that clinical oncologists correctly raise against therapists favoring unconventional methods," said Dr. Abel, "that they are unable to give scientific support to their claims, reflects on themselves" (3). Or, to put it in biblical terms, orthodox medicine should first remove the beam from its own eye before criticizing the mote in another's.

Braverman's modest proposal

"No disseminated neoplasm incurable in 1975 is curable today," oncologist Albert Braverman, M.D. wrote in 1991. For major kinds of cancer, "the rate and duration of remissions obtained for the more responsive tumors...have not improved and cures are rare." Yet "there has been no let-up in efforts devoted to trials of clinical chemotherapy, and in many of them the lack of benefit could have been predicted at the outset" (48). In a revealing portrait of what goes on inside the cooperative groups that decide on new treatment avenues, Braverman revealed:

"[A]t meetings of specific disease committees of cooperative groups there is a make-work atmosphere, with chairmen appealing to the audience to propose ideas for new regimens or drugs to study. These groups' raison d'être was not to invent questions, but to answer those arising from promising small (phase II) therapeutic trials. The phase II trials continue to appear, but, since virtually none are promising, the cooperative groups have become aimless."

He noted that "many medical oncologists recommend chemotherapy for virtually any tumor, with a hopefulness undiscouraged by almost invariable failure. The skills of many professionals are squandered upon these costly treatments." Braverman called on doctors to "scale back the whole chemotherapeutic enterprise" (48).

Four major biases

It has long been known that non-randomized studies are likely to give a biased assessment in favor of the experimental treatment and that physicians tend to act in a prejudiced manner unless suitably constrained by the methods of investigation (35). Advocates of new treatments tend to be overly optimistic about their own findings and to ardently want them to succeed. They thus consciously or unconsciously arrange the data to claim positive results (151).

There are several common errors in the interpretation of data that can make results appear better than they really are. Because of these widespread biases, patients and even doctors are often deceived into believing that a treatment offers more promise than it actually does.

Let us look at four of the major problems in cancer research: lead-time bias; stage migration; publication bias; and selection bias.

Lead-time bias

One of the most important errors made in interpreting data is "lead-time bias." The "lead-time" is essentially the length of time between the point at which a cancer is detected by new, sophisticated tests and the point at which it would formerly have been clinically detected by most doctors (260).

This problem was first explained in the late 1960s when mammography and other modern diagnostic techniques came into common use. A description of this bias was published in the *Journal of the National Cancer Institute* (118,190). Yet although it is universally acknowledged, this type of error is still committed over and over again.

What lead-time bias does is "extend the statistical length of a patient's survival without necessarily prolonging the duration of life" (15). Please study this sentence carefully! On paper, the patient appears to be surviving his or her cancer longer. But in actuality, there has been no real gain at all.

"Even if therapy is ineffectual," says Yale University School of Medicine's Prof. Alvan R. Feinstein, one of the pioneers of cancer biostatistics, "the period of survival will be increased" because of the "added time that is provided by the early, pre-symptomatic detection of the disease."

To repeat: the earlier the cancer is found, the longer the patient "survives." In actuality, however, no time has been added to the patient's survival. But on paper, there is great improvement.

Lead-time bias accounts for much of the illusory "improvement" seen over the last few decades in treating breast and other kinds of cancer. Patients are actually dying with the same regularity. But the statistics look a whole lot better.

These remarks of Feinstein were published in the *New England Journal of Medicine*, the most widely cited medical publication in the U.S. (119). Yet its startling conclusions are almost never taken into consideration by those who make public pronouncements concerning the alleged benefits of modern treatment.

THE PROBLEM OF FRAUD

Vast improvements in diagnostic techniques (such as MRIs, CAT scans, biochemical, and DNA markers), the intensification of screening (such as more mammograms or PSA tests for prostate cancer), self-observation (such as monthly breast self-examination), improvements in disease monitoring (such as the CEA test for colon cancer)— all can definitely result in earlier detection of the primary disease or the progression of metastases.

Survival may in some cases appear to improve greatly. But it is hasty and unjustifiable to attribute that improvement to chemotherapy.

Stage migration (Will Rogers phenomenon)

This phenomenon was first described in the *New England Journal of Medicine* in 1985 by Professor Feinstein (119). His brilliant analysis exposed another reason that much of the alleged progress in cancer treatment is probably spurious. Considering his prestigious position, and the venue of his article, one might think this too would be well known to scientists and to those who write about cancer "progress" in the media. But one rarely encounters any mention of this problem.

What happened was this: Feinstein and his colleagues set out to compare the course of treatment for New Haven lung cancer patients in the periods of 1953-64 and 1977. The "survival rates for the entire 1977 cohort and for subgroups...were higher than corresponding rates for the 1953-1964 cohort." Thus, the six-month survival of some lung cancer patients in the earlier period was 44 percent whereas in 1977 it had jumped to 55 percent. This is suspicious, because no major improvements had been made in the treatment of lung cancer in that period.

"We began to wonder, on further reflection," Feinstein recalled, "about the improved survival rates noted in the 1977 cohort." Certainly lead-time bias was at work, but there was something else going on, which he called *stage migration*. With better diagnostic techniques, lung-cancer patients' metastases were now being found in an "early" or "silent" condition. Thus, they were being staged differently, and placed into more advanced categories.

Patients with silent metastases were "migrating" from lower TNM stages into higher ones.

The net result was that more recent patients *appeared* to have survival rates that were considerably better than the 1953 to 1964 patients, "both for the entire group and for patients at each TNM stage." They had in fact "migrated" to higher stages of the disease.

In essence, "the[ir] migration would improve survival in the lower stages, because fewer patients with metastases would be assigned to them," Feinstein wrote. But, paradoxically, "migration would *also improve survival in the higher stages,* since the metastases in the newly added patients were silent rather than overt" (emphasis added).

"Although the total survival rate in the cohort would be unaffected, the stage-migration phenomenon could improve the survival rates in each of the constituent stages."

Stage migration led to an improvement in the prognosis for both early and more advanced stages. Early stages were being depleted of patients who had more advanced disease—hence figures for that stage appear better. At the same time, the more advanced group profits from the addition of patients who are less clinically advanced than they were in the past and have a relatively good prognosis.

Here was, truly, a win-win situation. Of course, nothing had really changed. People with lung cancer were dying at approximately the same depressing rate. But it sure looked better!

Feinstein credited this Zen-like paradox to the humorist-philosopher Will Rogers, who once said that "when the Okies left Oklahoma and moved to California, they raised the average intelligence level in both states."

By analogy, lung cancer patients "migrating" from earlier to later stages improved the statistics in both groups.

We can infer from this that the better modern medicine gets at detecting metastases, the more advanced the patients are likely to be classified upon discovery of their tumors. The same patient is more likely nowadays to be pigeonholed into a "worse" or "more advanced" category, when in fact nothing about his or her actual condition has really changed from a similar patient decades ago.

In the Yale-New Haven data, as we have seen, there was an 11 percent "increase" in six-month survival of some patients. Yet this was an illusion. Thanks to a shifting of patients, one could attribute improvement to treatment, which really was the result of statistical flukes.

Feinstein added, "These results are distressing because they suggest that the contemporary improvement of survival rates, at least among patients with lung cancer, is a statistical artifact."

It is also sobering to read, in America's premier medical journal:

"Results of this type in reports of post-treatment survival have served as a basis for the belief that modern therapy has substantially improved survival rates among patients with cancer" (119).

The clear implication is that the widespread belief in the effectiveness of some kinds of chemotherapy may be based on error and illusion.

Publication bias

This usually means that positive results on drugs are more readily published than negative ones. This is also called the "file drawer" bias, since negative results are more likely to remain locked up in a scientist's filing cabinet (99). This bias is also defined as "any tendency on the parts of investigators or editors to fail to publish study results on the basis of the direction or strength of the study findings" (100).

In a 1909 editorial in the *Boston Medical Journal,* a doctor complained: "We too commonly see references of 'so many successful cases,' with a certain inevitable emphasis on the word 'successful'....There is unquestionably a false emphasis in all such publications, tending to increase the reputation of the writer, but not render the public more secure" (15).

The first solid evidence of this bias did not emerge until 1986, however (343). Statisticians compared the results of two separate meta-analyses of chemotherapy for ovarian cancer. A meta-analysis is a paper in which the results of various smaller studies are pooled together to give the aggregate greater statistical reliability.

The particular question was whether combination chemotherapy was better than a single agent. When the statisticians considered the *published* studies, the result was positive. But when they considered *all* the trials that had been listed in a cancer trials registry, including those that for whatever reason had remained unpublished, "no statistically significant advantage of the combination chemotherapy was observed" (343).

The statisticians verified that the unpublished studies were of comparable quality to the published ones. The studies simply had been suppressed by their authors, perhaps because the results went against the dogma of combination chemotherapy.

In another study, authors of published randomized trials were asked about what other trials they had performed. It was found that they too had a great many studies tucked away in their file drawers. Once again, 55 percent of the published trials, but only 15 percent of unpublished studies, had statistically significant results favoring a new therapy (99).

In 1993, it was found by examining four studies performed at Johns Hopkins and Oxford Universities that there was "strong evidence of a positive association between statistically significant results and publication." It was the investigators themselves who barred publication. "The results of clinical trials should not be suppressed in this way," the authors mildly concluded (100).

One technical problem is that there is no central registry in the U.S.

of all on-going clinical trials (as there is, for example, in Spain). The result is that even scrupulously conducted meta-analyses may be compromised by the fact that not all studies (but only those submitted and selected for publication) are included. When unpublished trials are included, as they were in the above ovarian study, they may very well lose strength—or even lose statistical significance altogether.

In 1994, Dr. Abel commented, "More and more I have come to realize that publication bias is indeed a very strong source of bias in science, 'polluting' the published material" (5).

Selection bias

This bias originates in the rather obvious fact that healthier people tend to live longer than sickly ones. The bias arises if responders to therapy happen to be exactly those patients who would have lived longer anyway, whether or not they had received the experimental treatment.

How do scientists fall into this error? In some studies, people are started on the treatment not at the time of diagnosis, when they are symptom-free, but when they first begin to show signs of decline. But sometimes responders develop symptoms later than non-responders.

(In technical terms, they experience a significantly longer interval between their primary diagnosis and the time they entered the trial than the non-responders do.) This fact implies a slower growth rate of their tumors. In other words, the responders already had a better natural prognosis (a slower tumor growth rate) to begin with; not surprisingly, they lived longer (226). This is then chalked up to chemo.

Linguistic dodges

One also hears the word "cure" thrown around a great deal. In 1995, a consortium of cancer centers and drug companies including Amgen, Glaxo, and Zeneca launched a massive "Research Cures Cancer" advertising campaign, with public service announcements aired on TV stations and displayed in dioramas at U.S. airports (127).

For Webster, a cure is "something that corrects, heals, or permanently alleviates a harmful or troublesome situation," the "restoration of health from disease." In cancer the word "cure" has a peculiar import, different from its common meaning. To the cancer establishment, however, a cure is defined as a "five-year" or sometimes a "three-year" or even a "one-year" interval of survival from cancer. According to the orthodox book, *Everyone's Guide to Cancer Therapy*, "how [cure is] defined really depends on the kind of cancer being treated and on the individual patient" (104).

This conveniently provides a rubber ruler for chemotherapy's boosters to construct definitions of "cure" that serve their purposes. Let's say a patient has cancer and, through medical treatment, it goes into remission. Several months or years later there is a recurrence, and the cancer returns, more aggressive than it was before. Is that a cure? Not by any common meaning of the word. Yet that is precisely what happens in the field of cancer.

Oddly, a person can receive treatment for cancer, be clear of any signs or symptoms of cancer for five years, and be declared "cured." If the cancer then re-emerges, she can be in the paradoxical situation of being "cured" and dying of the disease at one and the same time.

Even if they are "cured," many people experience recurrence years after "successful" treatment. Many "cured" patients certainly live with the anxiety that their disease may return. Furthermore, if a treatment leaves the patient disabled, disfigured, incapacitated, or chronically exhausted (not to mention bankrupted) it is hardly reasonable to call that a "cure" in the normal sense of the term.

Even a top official of the ACS once admitted, "We really do not know what we mean by cure because there is a great difference between cure and long-term survival" (*New York Times*, 4/17/79).

What is more, if the treatment succeeds in giving you the very disease that it allegedly treats, it is difficult to call that a cure. Yet conventional cytotoxic drugs (and radiation) themselves cause cancer.

Equating "cure" with "five-year survival" can be highly misleading. Establishment sources argue that relative survival rates (i.e., figures adjusted for mortality in the normal population of the same age structure) remain fairly stable beyond five years. Twenty-year survival rates are said to be about 85 percent of five-year rates.

However, as Dr. Abel points out, "this information is obtained by improper pooling of disseminated and localized tumors" (3). For disseminated tumors, Abel says, "it is an enormous extenuation of reality." There's a big difference between localized tumors and those that have already spread. To know the real figures, one would have to break down the cases by whether or not they have spread, something that is not generally done.

Confusing tumor shrinkage with increased survival

There are, in addition, a number of linguistic loopholes that are employed in the cancer field. For instance, doctors sometimes try to equate "disease-free survival" with "absolute survival." But disease-free survival refers to an increase in the time that the patient is free of clinical cancer before a relapse occurs. Actual survival is increased lifespan, over what might have been expected if the patient had not taken the drug. Equating these two, or substituting one for the other is a nice bit of legerdemain that increases the "success" rate, without actually changing anything.

Another common linguistic dodge is to confuse tumor shrinkages with "success" in cancer treatment. The FDA defines a "response" in cancer as a reduction by 50 percent or more in all measurable tumors for 28 days or more. A complete response or remission (CR) is the total disappearance of all measurable tumors (the primary site tumor plus all detectable metastases). A partial response (PR) is the reduction by half or more of all measurable tumor. Such responses are the main yardstick in evaluating chemotherapeutic drugs.

The significance of this is that doctors routinely and regularly seek to bring about such "responses" and tell patients that this is a most desirable goal in their treatment. The reason for this is their belief that such "responses" correlate with increased survival.

However, this is not true, and constitutes one of the primary illusions in the field of cancer.

Thus, all is not as it seems in the evaluation of cancer drugs. Sometimes there is outright "cooking" of the experimental data. But more often, scientists fall victim to biases in the way they compile and present data to their peers and to the public. The net result almost always is to make chemotherapy appear to be far more effective than it really is for the vast majority of cancers.

CHAPTER SIX

Toxicity of Chemotherapy

~

"The next greatest misfortune to losing a battle
is to win such a victory as this."
—The Duke of Wellington, after the Battle of Waterloo (304)

CHEMOTHERAPY CAN HAVE ASTONISHING toxicity. In this chapter I shall review the general topic of toxicity, leaving a discussion of the specific properties of each drug for the *Appendices*. Lists of the FDA-approved cytotoxic drugs, and of common drug regimens, are also given in the *Appendices*.

Most of us are familiar with the usual side effects of chemotherapy: hair loss, mouth sores, nausea, and vomiting. The inexperienced reader might wonder what is so terrible about a few sores on the gums or a bout or two of the heaves. But language deceives us here. What are relatively minor symptoms when we encounter them in ordinary life can take on an entirely different dimension in patients on chemotherapy. Everyday experience hardly prepares us for the side effects experienced by some cancer patients. Their symptoms can be of an entirely different order of magnitude, and can even become lethal.

An oncology nurse's manual warns that cytotoxic agents pose a "significant risk" of damage to the skin, reproductive abnormalities, hematologic problems, and of liver and chromosomal lesions (232). And this is just to the health care workers preparing the drugs!

Nurses are instructed to protect themselves with long-sleeved gowns, face shields or goggles and latex surgical gloves, which should be changed every half hour. Unused drugs must be put in an impervious container labeled: "Caution: Biohazard." Nurses should also keep at the ready shoe covers; extra pairs of high-grade, extra-thick latex gloves; a disposable dustpan; plastic-lined towels; dessicant powder; disposable sponges; and a puncture-proof, leakproof container.

They are instructed to never eat, drink, smoke, or apply cosmetics in the drug-preparation area. With all this, they are warned that systemic absorption can occur when least expected. "You can accidentally inhale a drug while opening a vial, clipping a needle, expelling air from a syringe, or discarding excess drug that splashes," they are cautioned (232). Chemotherapy is serious business, indeed.

Hazards to public

These drugs may also pose a hazard to the general public, although this risk has been little explored. It is one thing to put surplus drugs into biohazard containers at the hospital. But more and more patients are receiving chemotherapy on an out-patient basis or at home. The drugs pose a risk to children and others who might inadvertently be exposed. And what happens when the patient uses the bathroom? When these highly toxic drugs (and their breakdown products or metabolites) are expelled in contaminated bodily wastes and fluids, they are often still in a dangerous form. They then usually find their way into the public sewage, where no special provisions have been made to dispose of them as toxic medical waste.

Ironically, they may become a source of cancer for future generations. The main toxicity, of course, is to the patients themselves, who swallow these drugs or have them injected or infused into various parts of their bodies.

Subtle effects

Not all the effects of the drugs are immediately obvious. During his wife's treatment for lung cancer, Robert Kotlowitz noted that drugs can have odd and subtle effects: "It doesn't take long for me to believe that the terrible, wild power of the chemo ruthlessly destroys what the tumor itself shuns. Taste is wiped out. Smell is both subverted and intensified. After the first chemo, the mere aroma of a boiled egg brings on agonizing nausea. The treatment is soon partner to the disease, a horrific paradox I keep to myself" (*New York Times*, 12/4/94).

Synthetic or natural?

We tend to think of cancer drugs as synthetic substances rationally conceived by scientists in the laboratory. Some are. But many cancer drugs are derived from empirically discovered natural poisons, such as paclitaxel (Taxol), vincristine, and cytarabine (ara-C). However, even when natural, such substances are still poisons that have been adapted for the purpose of killing cells, rather than for providing nutrition or gently boosting immunity.

Most drugs used against cancer share certain key characteristics. As the name "cytotoxic" implies, these drugs are poisonous, not just to cancer cells but to normal cells, as well. These are among the most dangerous substances ever introduced into the human body. Aside from the rigors of undergoing such an ordeal, chemotherapy is what is called a dose-limiting treatment. Bluntly put, that means that at a certain point doctors have to stop giving it or it may kill the patient.

There can be an Alice-in-Wonderland quality to scientific discussions of these effects. For instance, a 1995 report in the *Journal of Clinical Oncology* discussed the effects of a high-dose regimen called "ICE" (ifosfamide + carboplatin + etoposide) (120). This regimen has been used in metastatic breast cancer, non-Hodgkin's lymphoma, ovarian, and some other cancers.

The incidence of side effects was considerable. For example, 67 percent of the lower-dose patients had mucositis and 39 percent had enteritis. In the mid-range-dose patients, 50 percent suffered central nervous system (CNS) and lung complications. And in some of the higher-dose patients 61 percent suffered liver toxicity, 81 percent suffered ear damage, 70 percent suffered kidney toxicity, 92 percent suffered "adverse pulmonary events," while an extraordinary 94 percent suffered damage to their hearts (cardiotoxicity). There was also a case of coma and a "flaccid paralysis of all extremities" that "resolved over several months."

In all, 13 patients—or eight percent of the group—actually died of the effects of the drugs themselves, so-called "toxic deaths." Such deaths took place at almost every dose level. The immediate causes were widespread bacterial infections (sepsis), capillary leak syndrome, disseminated fungal infections (aspergillosis), bleeding inside the brain, and irreversible kidney failure. The underlying cause of death was ICE, and more specifically one component, ifosfamide, manufactured as IFEX by Bristol-Myers Squibb.

Well tolerated?

I have quoted these effects at some length not just for their own sake, but so that the reader can better appreciate the astonishing conclusion of this *Journal of Clinical Oncology* article. It reads:

"In summary, ICE is well tolerated, with acceptable hematopoietic [blood system related, ed.] side effects and predictable organ toxicity. Future studies that assess the activity of ICE...will be important to define its clinical usefulness" (120).

I had to read this over four or five times to convince myself that I was really reading a summation of the article in question. Perhaps one has to be an oncologist to share such an "ice-y" perspective.

The very journal that carried this report also ran a lead editorial entitled "Ifosfamide: Should The Honeymoon Be Over?" I thought that perhaps this would be an unprecedented condemnation of such harsh treatment. But the main point of the editorial was that ifosfamide has been oversold and that doctors should consider going back to its less expensive parent compound, cyclophosphamide (203).

Chemotherapy can cause cancer

Perhaps the strangest thing about chemotherapy is that many of these drugs themselves are carcinogenic. This may seem astonishing to the average reader—that cancer-fighting drugs themselves cause cancer. Yet this is an undeniable fact.

It is sometimes said that only the alkylating agents, such as busulfan, carmustine, and melphalan, are carcinogenic. But this is not true. The authoritative International Agency for Research on Cancer (IARC) has identified 20 single agents or regimens which cause cancer in humans, and about 50 more in which such effects are suspected (236,248). Many, but not all, of these are alkylating agents. The offending drugs include doxorubicin and streptozocin (toxic antibiotics used as cytotoxic agents), BCNU (a nitrosourea), as well as the various hormone-like products.

Perhaps the distinction between alkylating agents and other drugs in this regard is moot, since alkylating agents are prominently included in most of the regimens commonly used in cancer (see *Appendix B*).

To give just one example of carcinogenicity, doctors looked at one-year survivors of ovarian cancer from five randomized trials. The incidence rates for acute nonlymphocytic leukemia and for pre-leukemia were about 100 times more common in women who got the drug melphalan than in those who received no chemotherapy.

"The magnitude of these risks suggests that the drugs are causally related to leukemia," NCI epidemiologists cautiously concluded (97). However, they add, characteristically, that "the identification of a carcinogenic effect does not preclude its use for treatment in patients" (97). In other words, the fact that these drugs cause cancer is immaterial in the doctor's decision to administer these cytotoxic agents.

By combining various forms of chemotherapy, and then mixing these with radiotherapy, doctors further increase the risk. Even Dr. DeVita's orthodox textbook, *Cancer: Principles & Practice of Oncology*, concludes that "chemotherapy combinations can significantly raise the risk of secondary tumors, especially nonlymphocytic leukemias. The combination of lomustine, cyclophosphamide, and vincristine led to a leukemia incidence of 14 percent over 4 years after treatment. Nitrogen mustard, vincristine, prednisone, and procarbazine for the treatment of Hodgkin's disease yield leukemia rates up to 17 percent....Radiation further increases the risk of leukemia" (97).

Accelerating the cancer

These agents also can cause the formation of drug-resistant cells (20). They can thus paradoxically enhance the malignancy of the tumor and its ability to spread.

It is a common observation that patients sometimes seem to have an accelerated growth of cancer after receiving chemotherapy. This impression is often denigrated by oncologists. However, it is given credence from a study of patients who relapsed after treatment of breast cancer (186). Ninety-four out of 176 of these patients received chemotherapy after their relapse; the rest received endocrine treatment as a control.

There were favorable responses in 23 percent in the group that received the standard chemo protocol but in 47 percent of the patients in the *control* group. In addition, the disease began to progress after 9 weeks in the chemotherapy group, but in 17 weeks in the control patients (186). Clearly, after relapse, chemotherapy patients did worse.

In a 1987 scientific review of the topic, it was also found that cytotoxic drugs could promote the occurrence of metastases; suppress the immune system; damage the vascular system; and act directly and in a thoroughly unpredictable way on tumor cells (255).

Under such conditions, cancers can spread wildly (178).

Combination chemotherapy

In the "first generation" of chemotherapy, single agents, such as nitrogen mustard, methotrexate, and cyclophosphamide, were used alone. But in the second and third generations, following the examples of the treatment for Hodgkin's disease and childhood leukemia, single drugs were put together in complicated regimens, at high doses, in an attempt at overcoming drug resistance.

Since the 1970s, this use of such combination "cocktails" has now become a rock-solid guiding principle of chemotherapy. "For the last 10 years," two authors wrote in 1986, "it has been almost unquestioned dogma that combination chemotherapy is more effective than single-agent treatment in advanced breast cancer" (241). Yet, as they note, this does not generally result in increased survival for patients.

The development of "meaningful chemotherapy" is generally lauded in the history of cancer published by the NCI. However, the author of that 1979 history, the late Michael B. Shimkin, M.D., concluded that "its total contribution to the results [in cancer treatment, ed.] remains small" (342). He complained in the *New York Times* (8/6/85):

"We have gone on a binge of giving every cancer patient every possible chemotherapy, usually toxic cocktails made by mixing three or four different drugs....Chemotherapy is one of many areas where modern medicine has gone overboard."

Hormones and other agents are also commonly added. But because of the "dose-limiting" toxicity of these drugs (i.e., they may kill the patients if given too intensively), other drugs are needed to decrease the side effects. These are generally not given to ease the patient's plight but so that still higher doses can be given. These ancillary drugs themselves often turn out to have side effects of their own, such as bone pain, which in turn demands the use of other drugs, and so on (270).

The treatment of Hodgkin's disease, which is considered the model for most other cancers, illustrates how complicated combination chemotherapy has become. Drugs may include two regimens of four drugs each, used together or in alternating fashion. For non-Hodgkin's lymphoma, one of the protocols, called ProMACE-CYTABOM, includes the use of ten agents, including high-dose methotrexate, doxorubicin, and cyclophosphamide.

Perils of polypharmacy

In ancient and medieval times, such a proliferation of drugs was called "polypharmacy" (85). Even the FDA has recognized the dangers of complex combinations: "The combined effect of two or more drugs on the body can be very different from the action of each drug taken separately. Sometimes combining drugs can produce dangerous, even fatal, reactions. This is because each drug not only acts on the body but may act upon and increase the effect of other drugs, a condition known as potentiation" (*FDA Consumer Memo* 73-30, 1973).

Combinations also increase the development of sensitivities, increase side effects, confuse the clinical picture (202), and lead to "effects which might not have been expected if one had only considered the primary action of each individual drug" (194).

At the dawn of medical history, the Greek physician Hippocrates laid down the dictum, "First, do no harm." Poisons were of course well known at that time. Hippocrates was trying to teach doctors to avoid such poisonous substances and to focus their attention on safe medicine. This lesson has been ignored many times in the past.

In the eighteenth and nineteenth centuries, doctors made a virtual cult out of poisonous drugs like calomel (mercurous chloride), giving them on almost every occasion. This contributed to a massive patient rebellion, until finally doctors were forced to give up on their favorite remedy (85). "Polychemotherapy" is polypharmacy in modern garb. It may take an even greater rebellion on the part of patients and health workers before medical leaders will stop encouraging the use of toxic drugs in situations where they do far more harm than good.

CHAPTER SEVEN

A Multi-Billion-Dollar Business

AROUND THE WORLD, CHEMOTHERAPY HAS become a common medical procedure. In fact, it has become unusual to find a cancer patient who is not given chemotherapy or urged, sometimes in the strongest possible terms, to take chemical treatments for cancer.

"The majority of patients receive some form of...toxic therapy before death," Dr. Abel wrote in 1990, and "in virtually all cases such treatment is taken into consideration" (3).

"We feel that antineoplastic [i.e., cytotoxic] therapy should be offered to as many patients as possible," wrote a group of American doctors (182). Former NCI director Vincent DeVita, M.D., regards virtually all patients with metastatic or recurrent disease as candidates for chemotherapy (95).

In breast, colon, lung, ovarian, and many other kinds of cancer, the use of chemotherapy, sometimes together with surgery or radiation, has become almost routine. In many countries, chemotherapy has become a matter of health care policy. The U.S. government suggests that "all newly diagnosed patients with breast cancer may appropriately be considered as candidates for one of the numerous ongoing clinical trials..." (278). These often utilize combinations of powerful drugs.

Size of marketplace

How many people actually receive chemotherapy each year? The short but amazing answer is: No one is keeping track. A common estimate is 300,000. But by my calculations the true number is closer to one million people in the U.S. alone.

One prime source of information is the National Cancer Data Base's (NCDB), *Annual Review of Patient Care—1994*. This report was prepared by the American Cancer Society (ACS) and the American College of Surgeons Commission on Cancer (355). The NCDB deals with six of the most common solid tumors of adults: gastric, colon and rectal, pancreatic, breast, ovarian, and prostate.

These types of cancer represent about 600,000 cases of the disease per year. Of these cases, we learn that 175,000 are likely to receive chemotherapy as part of their hospital treatment for cancer.

Since 600,000 represents about half of the new U.S. cases we can extrapolate from this that about 350,000 U.S. patients receive chemotherapy each year. I think this is where a commonly cited figure of 300,000 recipients per year comes from.

But it is important to note that these NCDB figures apply only to *in-hospital admissions*. What about the increasing number of patients whose oncologists or primary care physicians prescribe some form of chemotherapy outside the context of hospital admissions? We do not know. But it is a reasonable guess that for every patient who receives chemotherapy while a hospital in-patient, another receives it in the out-patient department, in the doctor's office, in the hospice, or at home. Thus, the actual figure in 1991 was probably at least 700,000.

What has happened since then? As we shall see, chemotherapy sales worldwide are increasing at double-digit rates. Assuming that the number of patients is also growing by double digits, the actual figure for chemotherapy recipients should be approximately one million patients per year. And these are just the U.S. patients.

Expenses to patients

And what of the cost? Such treatments can be very expensive, running into the tens, or even hundreds, of thousands of dollars per patient. No firm figures are available yet, but we can infer the amount from these facts gleaned from medical journals and newspapers:

• In 1995, the patient's cost for a course of the drug ifosfamide was placed at $3,925, with another $5,000 to $6,000 for hospitalization, for a total of about $10,000 for a five-day course (203). That's for one drug in a multi-drug regimen that often also includes the drugs cisplatin and etoposide. Nor does that $10,000 include the cost of treating any of the side effects that may accompany the use of these drugs (120).

• *The New York Times* estimated the standard drug treatment for breast cancer as costing between $5,000 and $25,000 (211).

• The late Dr. Charles Moertel of the Mayo Clinic said that six months' therapy at manufacturer's recommended doses are $7,000 for carboplatin and from $6,500 to $75,000 for alpha interferon. "These prices," he said, "are just for the drug alone" and do not include supportive care that often runs into additional tens of thousands of dollars.

• Moertel also pointed to the "astronomical price tags on new cancer drugs." He reviewed a claim for a single individual for nearly $750,000 for drug treatment, most of it for "off-label" uses of drugs (i.e., uses that lacked sufficient evidence of effectiveness to get FDA approval).

• Costs soar when bone marrow transplantation (BMT) is involved. This procedure allows doctors to give extra-high doses of radiation and/or chemotherapy and is becoming increasingly common. Over 1,000 American women with breast cancer received it in 1994 outside of approved clinical trials. BMT costs $60,000 to $200,000 (211). A man wrote to the *New York Times* that if Blue Cross/Blue Shield did not pay for the procedure, "I will be forced to sell my house, borrow from friends and relatives, and mortgage my children's future" (331).

• In 1995, the *New York Times* also carried the story of a woman who was treated for chronic granulocytic leukemia from the fall of 1993 until her death in January, 1995. Her treatments included chemotherapy, full-body radiation, and a bone marrow transplantation. The *Times* mentions that her "unpaid medical bills" totaled $600,000 (22).

A third way of assessing the dimensions of the chemotherapy marketplace is to look at worldwide sales. A market intelligence company, Frost & Sullivan, has kept track of this over the last few years. This report shows that the world cancer therapeutics market reached $8.6 billion in 1995 and is expected to reach $13.8 billion by 1999.

Cancer Therapeutics Market Revenue Forecasts (World) 1989-1999

Year	Revenues ($ million)	Revenue Growth Rate (%)
1989	3,104.6	–
1990	3,531.2	13.7
1991	4,356.8	23.4
1992	5,808.0	33.3
1993	6,710.4	15.5
1994	7,514.9	12.0
1995	8,590.6	14.3
1996	9,798.8	14.1
1997	10,979.8	12.1
1998	12,300.1	12.0
1999	13,790.4	12.1

Compound Annual Growth Rate (1992-1999): 13.1 percent
Note: All figures are rounded off. Source: Frost & Sullivan Market Intelligence.

This amazing double-digit growth has been fueled by introduction of what it calls "premium-priced products" on a world scale. Such candor is not for public consumption: these reports on the cancer marketplace are priced at several thousand dollars apiece; but useful summaries were made available to us by Frost & Sullivan (131).

The U.S., which is the largest manufacturer, also remains the largest national market for cancer therapeutics. Frost & Sullivan researchers broke sales down into three general areas: cytotoxic and hormonal treatments; cytokines, like the interferons and interleukins; anti-emetics to reduce nausea and vomiting caused by the above.

Largest manufacturers

According to the Pharmaceutical Manufacturers Association (PMA), the number of member companies developing cancer drugs increased from 56 in 1988 to 65 in 1991.

Some of the largest manufacturers are Adria, Bristol-Myers Squibb Oncology, Burroughs-Wellcome, Merck, Roche, and Upjohn. All such drugs have been patented, or otherwise monopolized, by these pharmaceutical companies. They are usually expensive and profitable. Sophisticated full-color ads fill the pages and help fund the major cancer journals in which such drugs are often discussed.

Since the 1980s, the number of drugs in development doubled, from 65 to 126. Four new companies also entered the market in the 1990s: Sandoz, Glaxo Holdings, SmithKline Beecham, and Amgen.

Globalization is also increasing, here as in the rest of the massive pharmaceutical industry. This is logical, since it increases so-called economies of scale. Consolidation is also occurring, through the formation of subsidiaries, joint ventures, mergers, and strategic alliances.

It is noteworthy that while chemotherapy's absolute sales are up year by year, its projected *share* of the overall cancer marketplace slowly declines. For example, while chemotherapy represented 90.3 percent of revenues in 1989, by 1995 this is projected to slip to about two-thirds of the market. This is because the sale of cytokines (such as interferons, interleukins, etc.) will soon represent a substantial portion of the market. While these are natural in origin, the way they are prepared and given makes them akin to toxic chemotherapy.

Census Bureau data

Another way of grasping the scope of the huge chemotherapy marketplace is through the Census of Manufactures of the U.S. Bureau of the Census (374). These reports similarly reveal the enormous growth in the cancer marketplace over the last two decades.

For the broad category "pharmaceutical preparations affecting neoplasms, the endocrine system, and metabolic diseases, for human use," there was a doubling of U.S. shipments between 1987 and 1992—from $1.9 billion to $3.8 billion. For cytotoxic drugs, the total of U.S. shipments was $893 million in 1992, the last year available for analysis.

This is a fraction of the Frost & Sullivan figure because the Census only gives the value of shipments from U.S. factories. Drugs produced by U.S. plants abroad or even in Puerto Rico are not included in this figure, nor—since these are strictly U.S. figures—are sales by foreign companies, such as ICI, Glaxo, Sandoz, etc., although in this era of globalization such distinctions are becoming increasingly meaningless.

Hospital discharges
One can also look at hospital admissions and discharges. The latest reports from the Agency for Health Care Policy and Research (AHCPR) are dated 1994; however, they report on the year 1987 (7). In that year, there were over 2.2 million discharges of cancer patients from U.S. hospitals. The total in-hospital billing for these patient visits was $13.9 billion which, according to the AHCPR, represented 9.8 percent of the total U.S. hospital bill for that year.

This was about double the estimate of $6.4 billion made for the year 1975 (168) and $7.2 billion made just two years later (181). By far the most costly malignant diseases nationwide were cancers of the digestive tract ($2.8 billion), followed by those of the respiratory tract ($1.5 billion), and the female reproductive organs ($1.2 billion).

Let us return for a moment to the 9.8 percent figure given above for cancer's share of the U.S. health bill. This is important, for not long before it was estimated that only "about 5 percent of the resources within the health care sector are used to treat, prevent or mitigate the effects of cancer" (200). Assuming this was at one time correct, the cost of treating cancer has risen rapidly compared to other diseases and conditions. It is claimed that each hospital admission for cancer now generates an extraordinary two to three times the billings of a typical non-cancer admission (249).

Financial impact
Using that 9.8 percent yardstick, we can estimate the financial impact of cancer on American society: since the U.S. health bill is around $900 billion, the direct cost of cancer is about *$90 billion.*

For the last few years the ACS and NCI have estimated cancer's overall U.S. cost at $104 billion, although they apportion this figure in a way that seriously underestimates the amount of money being spent on cancer treatment.

Thus, their estimate for direct (treatment-related) costs is only $35 billion, with the rest divided between the costs of morbidity (lost productivity) and mortality. However, since ACS itself says that "cancer accounts for about ten percent of the total cost of disease in the U.S." and that "an estimated $900 billion will be spent on health care this year in the United States," it is hard to avoid a direct cost figure of $90 billion (11).

Notional patient benefit year

Finally, we can ask what is the actual cost of increasing survival through chemotherapy? Economists call this its "economic efficiency." Astonishingly, there are few studies that address this obvious question. Bengt Jönsson, a Professor of Health Economics at the Stockholm School of Economics, Sweden, has reported that he could only find a single study based on a randomized trial which provided a complete cost-benefit and cost-utility analysis of chemotherapy (200).

Of course, costs vary widely from one diagnosis and one case to another. Some cases of acute myeloid leukemia, for example, cost three times as much as other cases, depending on the age group, and whether or not the cancer had gone into remission.

Obviously, if the treatment "works" then it is worth a lot more than if it doesn't. That is why economists have devised a new measure for evaluating health care called the *notional patient benefit year* (NPBY) cost (317). In cancer, this essentially refers to the cost that society pays for each year of cancer-free survival attained by treatment. NPBY is especially useful in seeing the relative values of different treatments. Dr. Jönsson gives some typical figures (200):

Relative Values of Cancer Treatments

Treatment	NPBY costs (US $)
Surgery and radiotherapy for stage 1 testicular cancer	$ 125
Cytotoxic chemotherapy for metastatic teratoma	172
Tamoxifen for advanced breast cancer	593
A study of cisplatin and methotrexate in bladder cancer	24,960
Chemotherapy for metastatic non-small-cell lung cancer with cyclophosphamide, doxorubicin and etoposide	28,080
Chemotherapy for advanced, previously treated, non-small-cell lung cancer with vindesine, etoposide and cisplatin	174,720

Where chemotherapy is truly effective, such as in the treatment of testicular cancer, it "tends to be a cheap alternative in relation to the outcome," says Jönsson. But in most cases it is a very "costly treatment." Thus, patients (and/or third-party insurers) must pay almost $175,000 for one year of cumulative extra survival time for non-small-cell lung cancer patients. But that does not mean that many individual patients actually have increased survival of a year due to chemotherapy. It is patients in the aggregate who pay this price, prorated to their own survival. Dr. Jönsson suggested that this type of analysis can be used to provide patients with information on the actual cost of conventional treatment. The patient should be given "the opportunity to choose between alternatives rather than to try to find the one and only 'best' alternative for all patients." Cost is not everything but neither is it irrelevant when the patient is probably paying part of the costs of treatment and trying to help make treatment decisions.

Drug company influence on research centers

It has long been my contention that the leaders of the cancer war are influenced, either consciously or unconsciously, by their intimate involvement with drug makers and their own financial interests (269).

The marketing of toxic drugs lies at the heart of the "war on cancer." For example, in one study, the cost of the drugs was 55 percent of total treatment cost for small-cell lung cancer (360). One company, Bristol-Myers Squibb, is particularly influential. Bristol-Myers Squibb spends more than one billion dollars per year on research and employs 4,000 scientists and support personnel (50). It holds patents on more than a dozen drugs approved by the FDA for the treatment of cancer; this accounts for almost half of the chemotherapy sales in the world (269).

Bristol-Myers Squibb also creatively influences cancer research. It gives out awards, lectures, and grants of many kinds. It pays for updates to orthodox cancer textbooks, and supports research and "data management" of clinical studies on its patented agents (120). Other cancer drug companies do the same.

Drug companies, again with Bristol-Myers Squibb in the forefront, occupy a very strong position at Memorial Sloan-Kettering:
• James D. Robinson III, the Chairman of the MSKCC Board of Overseers and Managers, is a director of Bristol-Myers Squibb.
• Richard L. Gelb, Vice-Chairman of the MSKCC board, is chairman of the board of Bristol-Myers Squibb.
• Richard M. Furlaud, MSKCC board member, retired in 1994 as president of Bristol-Myers Squibb. He has also been a director of the Pharmaceutical Manufacturers Association.
• Benno C. Schmidt, Honorary co-chairman of MSKCC, is the founder and board member of Genetics Institute, a Massachusetts-based company that manufactures drugs for the cancer marketplace. He is also a director of Gilead Sciences (which makes cancer-related drugs) (19); Matrix and Vertex Pharmaceuticals. He received the Bristol-Myers Award for distinguished service to cancer research in 1979.
• Paul A. Marks, M.D., the President and CEO of MSKCC, is a

director of Pfizer, which manufactures cancer-related drugs. He is also on the board of National Health Labs and of Life Technologies.

Aggressive pro-chemo stance

Under their leadership, MSKCC continues its aggressively pro-chemotherapy stance, and has eschewed almost all nontoxic alternatives. This has had major implications for the international direction of cancer treatment. In some cases, individual board members have advanced their own careers and fortunes. These facts are generally unknown to the average person who puts $20 in an envelope to help the war against cancer, to the patient who receives the chemotherapy, and to some of the doctors who administer the drugs.

However, it is certainly legitimate to ask, "To whose benefit is the war on cancer being fought?" Why do doctors who must know of the lack of efficacy of their drugs continue to give it?

Dr. Martin F. Shapiro explained in the *Los Angeles Times* that while "some oncologists inform their patients of the lack of evidence that treatments work...others may well be misled by scientific papers that express unwarranted optimism about chemotherapy. Still others respond to an economic incentive. Physicians can earn much more money running active chemotherapy practices than they can providing solace and relief...to dying patients and their families" (340).

The war on cancer is big business and chemotherapy has become a major profit center for hospitals, doctors, and drug companies.

By 1995, even the editor of the *Journal of the American Medical Association*, George D. Lundberg, complained at an NIH meeting: "Efforts by those with vested interests to influence decision-makers to use their power are ever more creative; efforts by manufacturers to influence publications so that they position their products in as favorable a light as possible are pervasive and frequently well-disguised... [it's] a marvelous opportunity for rampant deceit. So much money is there to be made that ethical principles can be overrun, sometimes in a stampede to get at physicians and prescribers" (239).

Did you hear this on the evening news? Of course not. Nobody in a position of authority will tell the public that toxic drugs are sometimes inappropriately administered because it is financially beneficial for a great many people to do so. Quite the opposite. At all costs, the public must be convinced that chemotherapy works, and that it is in their best interest to be quiet, take their medicine, and leave the thinking on such abstruse matters to those who wear white coats.

In my opinion, patients will do so at their peril.

CHAPTER EIGHT

Chemo for Particular Cancers

"Whether any of the common cancers can be cured by chemotherapy has yet to be established."
—John Cairns, *Scientific American*, Nov. 1985 (60)

GRANDIOSE CLAIMS ARE OFTEN made for chemotherapy. It is my contention, however, that chemotherapy is basically ineffective in the vast majority of cases in which it is given. Nor is there any immediate prospect that it will soon become much more effective.

Of course, we have shown that chemotherapy *does* lead to meaningful life extension in some relatively rare kinds of cancer. But the astonishing thing is that most of that progress was achieved before the start of the war on cancer. In October, 1971, in fact, Dr. Gordon Zubrod, a leader of the National Cancer Institute, presented a list of malignancies which were already highly responsive to chemotherapy (408):

Cancers Responsive to Chemotherapy By 1971

Disease	*Therapy*
Burkitt's lymphoma	Cyclophosphamide
Choriocarcinoma	Methotrexate, Dactinomycin
Acute Lymphocytic Leukemia	Combinations of Drugs
Hodgkin's Disease	Combinations of Drugs
Lymphosarcoma	Combinations of Drugs
Embryonal Testicular Cancer	Combinations of Drugs
Wilms' Tumor	Surgery + Drugs
Ewing's Sarcoma	Surgery + Drugs
Rhabdomyosarcoma	Surgery + Drugs
Retinoblastoma	Surgery + Drugs

After almost a quarter century of effort, and the expenditure of over $50 billion on cancer research, what has been the result? The list today is almost identical to what it was 25 years ago! Has chemotherapy been shown to be really effective against any of the common, solid tumors of adults, which are responsible for about 90 percent of cancer deaths every year? To answer that question soberly and scientifically we must at least see some compelling direct or indirect evidence that the treatment results in significant increased survival. And if it doesn't do that, can it improve the cancer patient's quality of life?

The astonishing fact is that these questions are not even asked, much less answered, for the majority of cancers. For all the different types of advanced adult carcinomas, for example, comparisons against good supportive care have been performed only for carcinomas of the lung, stomach, and pancreas. And the results were entirely negative in the case of stomach and pancreatic cancer (3). We shall examine the "positive" results in lung cancer below.

As for the many other kinds of carcinoma, one may well ask whether chemotherapy is of any survival benefit at all. The brief answer is that, with a few exceptions, it is not, as far as evidence from clinical trials can tell us.

A word about organization: in this chapter I shall first discuss four common types of adult cancers in which chemotherapy is often given and for which some claims can reasonably made for its effectiveness. These are cancers of the breast, especially adjuvant treatment after surgery for stages I and II; colon, especially Dukes' C; small-cell lung cancer; and ovarian cancer.

These are followed by an alphabetized overview of almost 50 types of cancer, for most of which any claims of positive effects are almost impossible to document.

Breast

In the U.S., the treatment of breast cancer has now become the hub of the entire cancer controversy. In 1993, breast cancer activists marched on Washington, delivering a petition with 2.6 million signatures, demanding more research money for this disease. Much of that money has gone for further research on chemotherapy.

Death rates for breast cancer vary greatly around the world from 4.6 per 100,000 in China to 28.7 in England and Wales—an almost sevenfold difference. Denmark, Ireland, Luxembourg, and New Zealand also have high rates. The rate in the United States is 22.4, while in Japan it is 6.3, the lowest by far in the industrial world (10).

Among U.S. women, the death rate from breast cancer is second only to lung cancer; in Germany it is first. One in eight American women is now slated to develop breast cancer in her lifetime. In the U.S. in 1995, there will be an estimated 182,000 new cases, and 46,240 patients will die. While predominantly a female disease, 1,000 such cases occur each year in men, with approximately 240 deaths (11).

Breast cancer is primarily treated by surgery. However, the use of chemotherapy is increasing at almost every stage. There was nearly a doubling of drug use in the years between 1985-86 and 1991.

Treatment of Breast Cancer in U.S. Hospitals

Year	Surg. & Chemo	Surg. Rad. & Chemo	Chemo Alone*	Total
1985/86	14.8	7.2	1.7	23.7
1991	24.4	14.6	1.6	40.6

*Chemotherapy alone includes hormonal therapy. Figures are percentages of hospital in-patients receiving treatment by the above methods.

Thus, over 40 percent of women were receiving chemotherapy as part of their in-hospital treatment of breast cancer in 1991. The number is probably higher today. Plus, as we have indicated before, such statistics do not tell us about women receiving chemotherapy outside of the in-hospital setting.

The NCDB report states that survival correlates with the stage and histologic grade of the tumor, the patient's age, ethnic background, and income. However, what it does not state is whether there was any correlation at all between increased survival and the aggressiveness of the treatment, especially the use of drugs.

Treatment varies depending on a number of things, but especially on the tumor stage.

The stages of breast cancer

0: Non-invasive lobular in situ and ductal carcinoma in situ. These are small tumors, generally curable with a wide excision of the tumor. Positive nodes are rare.

I: Tumor is 3/4 of an inch (2 cm) or less in size. No evidence of spread to nearby lymph nodes or distant sites.

IIa: This stage designates either a small primary lesion, less than 3/4 of an inch (2 cm) with positive axillary (armpit) lymph nodes, or a larger primary lesion without positive nodes.

IIb: This suggests a primary lesion between 3/4 and 2 inches (2-5 cm) and positive axillary nodes, or a large tumor greater than 2 inches, without positive axillary nodes.

IIIa: A big tumor over 2 inches (5 cm) with involvement of the axillary lymph nodes on the same side as the tumor.

IIIb: Large tumor, with involvement of lymph nodes of the chest or extension of tumor into chest wall or involvement of the skin.

IV: Distant metastases (e.g., to bone, liver, or lung) or skin and chest wall involvement beyond the breast area.

Hormone receptivity

Some breast tumors are particularly responsive to circulating sex hormones, especially estrogen. The growth of some tumors is stimulated by the female hormone estrogen, which makes them grow more rapidly. These are called estrogen receptor positive tumors, abbreviated ER+. This is a biochemical marker found on cancer cells. Those tumors that do not have that marker are called estrogen receptor negative, or ER–.

Patients also respond quite differently depending on their age and particularly whether or not they have experienced menopause, which usually occurs in one's late 40s or early 50s. (Sometimes menopause is triggered or induced by treatment.)

The adjuvant treatment of breast cancer

The NCI's on-line PDQ system advises that "all newly diagnosed patients with breast cancer may appropriately be considered as candidates for one of the numerous ongoing clinical trials"(278). Most writers on this topic agree that, statistically, some patients can have their lives extended by taking such treatment. Many questions remain:

• How many women are really benefited?
• How many receive treatment who do not need it or will not benefit?
• Is there harm in giving this treatment to large numbers of women?

There is evidence that adjuvant chemotherapy somewhat reduces the incidence of recurrence and extends survival for a small percentage of the women who are given it. Since no one knows who will benefit and who will not, the rest have to take it with no benefit to themselves. But all who take it must suffer both the short- and long-term side effects, which include the possibility of "toxic deaths" and of initiating or promoting second cancers.

The initial conventional treatment for early-stage breast cancer is surgery. If this is a lumpectomy, it is advised that the woman also have local irradiation to the site of the tumor. The great majority of such early stage patients will have no recurrence of their tumors. They will live 5, 10, even 20 or more years without any further problem. For all intents and purposes these patients are "cured," at least by the conventional definitions of the word "cure."

Why then give all these women adjuvant chemotherapy? Because their doctors believe that the various organs of their bodies harbor secret nests of metastatic breast cancer cells.

There is something strange about this sudden conversion of the oncology profession to the theory of "micrometastases." Not long ago, these same doctors dogmatically held the opposite view. For 200 years, from the time of John Hunter (1728-1793) till about 1980, the philosophy of breast cancer as a localized disease held sway. Hunter ardently hoped that cancer was not a "constitutional" disease. That "would be terrible, indeed," he wrote, "as we have no specific nor even a palliative for it..." (342).

The Halsted radical mastectomy was the outcome of such thinking, and it became dogma that breast cancer was a surgical disease. "We got it all," became the watchword of breast cancer treatment. The heresy at that time was that breast cancer was a constitutional illness.

What happened? Chemo.

Now, everyone points to the fact that breast cancers have almost invariably spread by the time they are operated upon. "It is generally accepted that at the time of presentation early breast cancer is a systemic disease in the majority of patients," Alan J. Wilson and colleagues wrote in 1986 (394). This is a typical view.

Although this sounds pretty "holistic," there is something amiss with this view. As Steve Austin, N.D. and Kathy Hitchcock, M.S.W. explain in their 1994 book, *Breast Cancer:*

"In reality, though, the conventional medical paradigm still doesn't treat breast cancer as systemic; it continues to view the disease as a group of microscopic, localized problems" (26).

Holistic thinkers tend to see cancer as a generalized problem that becomes localized, whereas conventional doctors see it as a localized problem that becomes generalized. A person with a truly holistic approach would not view the damage that chemotherapy inflicts on the defense systems of the body, or the well-being of the patient, as trivial.

Micrometastasis hypothesis

It is true that small growths, called micrometastases, have been found in the bodies of breast cancer patients; but the inferences drawn from this fact may be erroneous. As Austin and Hitchcock write:

"The conclusion that chemotherapy is the only or best way to deal with these pockets of cancer (or that the micrometastases will necessarily turn into life-threatening cancer) is still speculative. In a sense, we can say that this approach stands on about as much solid ground as did the old Halsted radical mastectomy theory" (26).

The European (EORTC) reviewers go out of their way to call this micrometastasis theory "hypothetical" and "putative." Yet it is this very theory that justifies—in fact, practically demands—the use of a systemic treatment, in this case adjuvant chemotherapy, in the treatment of breast cancer. This has led to an enormous increase in the use of drugs—usually the CMF regimen in premenopausal women, as well as tamoxifen in the postmenopausal patients.

In fact, it is absurd to say that because of the existence of micro-metastases breast cancer is never really cured. For example, in the years 1974 to 1986, before adjuvant chemotherapy began in earnest, the five-year survival rate for localized breast cancer among U.S. women of all races and ages was 91 percent (323). Thus, while the micrometastasis theory might be technically true, *at least nine out of ten women with early stage breast cancer will not have a recurrence once their tumor is excised.* The great majority of such women are simply "cured" by appropriate surgery. And that tenth woman will not necessarily be "cured" by chemo.

Yet, today, almost all these women are being urged to take highly toxic chemotherapy for up to a year or more. How did this situation arise?

The first trials

Chemotherapy really became established in the U.S. with the formation of the Cancer Chemotherapy National Service Center of the National Institutes of Health (NIH) in 1954 (148). The first randomized trial of chemotherapy for breast cancer was begun by this center in 1957 (122). This program eventually became the National Surgical Adjuvant Project for Breast and Bowel Cancer, or NSABP. It was headed, from the first, by Bernard Fisher, M.D., the same man who was ousted from his leadership of the program in 1994 for mishandling the rampant fraud in this program.

Fisher was first author on an early trial of the drug thiotepa, and over the years on many subsequent studies upholding the value of adjuvant chemotherapy in breast cancer.

In that first trial, after surgery, patients received either a short course of thiotepa or a placebo. There were 1,465 patients enrolled in this trial. According to the European (EORTC) review, "thiotepa had no effect on the number of treatment failures or deaths at 5 or 10 years..." (394). According to Dr. Gerald Moore of Roswell Park, after four years thiotepa "seems to be most effective as an adjuvant to the pre-menopausal patient with lymph node metastases" (267). Irwin Bross, Ph.D. was biostatistician for these trials and the study was centralized in his Department of Biostatistics at Roswell Park Memorial Institute for Cancer Research in Buffalo, New York (54).

In a 1994 book he gave a candid inside view of these early adjuvant trials. In his opinion, the first studies in the 1960s had a positive result. It showed that "an ablative therapy...the adjuvant chemotherapy used in the first study (thiotepa) had produced the first improved survival in the treatment of breast cancer."

These modest results were achieved, however, not by using aggressive chemotherapy to kill every last cancer cell but by decreasing the amount of hormones in the cancer's environment—what is called chemical ablation. It was an approach pioneered by Dr. Thomas Dao, innovative head of Roswell Park's breast surgery department.

This was "the first major advance in the treatment of breast cancer in more than half a century....Ironically," Bross added, this discovery "did not lead to further exploration of the ablative approach; in fact, it led to virtual suppression of this promising research line!"

Oncologists opted instead to increase the dosages and complexities of chemotherapy, to reach the kinds of regimens we see today. This may explain why textbooks virtually ignore the mild thiotepa trial and claim that the first randomized trials "based on the modern techniques" date from a decade later (97).

More toxic treatment

In that second trial, conducted between 1972 and 1975, NSABP tested a protocol called B-05 in 370 node-positive patients, in which some women received placebo and others received another relatively mild drug called L-PAM. After two years, there seemed to be an overall advantage in disease-free survival of ten percent in the L-PAM treated group. In a sub-group analysis, it was found there was a "disease-free survival" advantage of 22 percent among the patients who were younger than 50 years, but a negligible four percent in those over 50.

It is extremely important to bear in mind that "disease-free survival" is not the same thing as overall or absolute survival. Disease-free survival is essentially a measure of the time until recurrence; one can die at exactly the same time, yet have a wonderful increase in "disease-free survival." In my opinion, it is a confusing and largely meaningless parameter of improvement. It tells you how long you will live without signs of the disease; it does not tell you if you will actually live any longer than you would have if you had not taken the treatment.

This second NSABP study was also marked by what may, in retrospect, have been statistical irregularities. For example, 22 of the patients were bumped from the analysis as the trial progressed. Such exclusions could have affected the outcome and statistical significance of the results.

British trials

Meanwhile, there was activity in Europe, especially England, to test adjuvant treatments. Between 1975 and 1979, the so-called Guy's-Manchester Trial attempted to repeat the second NSABP trial. After about four years they found no overall significant difference in their relapse-free survival (330). At that time U.S. advocates of chemotherapy accused the British of administering "inadequate treatment." This now seems unlikely, because the British patients suffered as much damage to their bone marrow (myelosuppression) as those in the U.S. trial—a rather grim marker for the "adequate" application of any treatment.

The British scientists concluded that L-PAM has "no place...as an adjuvant to mastectomy in routine clinical practice" (330).

The Italian bombshell

Then, in 1976, came a dramatic report from the National Cancer Institute of Milan, Italy of an alleged major breakthrough using a combination of drugs as an adjuvant treatment for early stage breast cancer (41). This trial, begun by Gianni Bonadonna, M.D. and colleagues in 1973, randomized 391 node-positive women to either no treatment or to 12 cycles of cyclophosphamide + methotrexate + fluorouracil (CMF) for over 1 year. Initial reports spoke excitedly of a doubling of survival time. Because of this study, CMF became the most commonly used form of adjuvant chemotherapy for premenopausal women with stages I or II breast cancer.

After nine years, the results shrank to far more modest proportions: an increase of 12 percent in relapse-free survival and 11 percent in overall survival. It is noteworthy that survival benefits were entirely in the younger, premenopausal group of patients, and not at all in those who were postmenopausal (43).

But was it true? There were clouds over the Milan data: patients who were unable to complete the rather arduous CMF therapy were withdrawn from the treatment and then not included in the subsequent randomizations. By the end, 29 patients had been withdrawn in this way (41). In fact, the only patients to benefit were those who could tolerate a "full or nearly full dose." These represented only 17 percent of the total, according to a trenchant critique by H. Vorherr of Albuquerque, NM (385). Often, such treatment "dropouts" have a worse prognosis, which may be what led them to withdraw from the trial in the first place. But removing them from consideration in the treatment group made the results look better than they really were.

This type of exclusion of patients tips the balance toward the treatment arm, "thus wrecking the very reason for randomization," according to Dr. Alan J. Wilson writing in the EORTC review (394).

It may be noteworthy that Dr. Bonadonna, often in the past an ardent spokesperson for chemotherapy, himself has become more reserved about the application of such adjuvant treatments than some of his followers. In 1992, he wrote about women who are ER+ and/or have stage I breast tumors:

"The vast majority of these women can be spared chemotherapy" (44). But, of course, he cannot now stop the momentum that he put into motion with his 1976 study.

The Milan studies had a catalytic effect on chemotherapy, especially for breast cancer. Although a 1980 NIH meeting concluded that the results were only proven useful in the comparatively small group of premenopausal women with involved axillary nodes (279), the Milan results gave a green light to all sorts of applications beyond this relatively small group. In fact, soon afterwards, there was a "premature abandonment of no-treatment control groups in the majority of subsequent trials of cytotoxic chemotherapy" (394).

This was highly significant. It was no longer even "ethical" to run studies that asked the question of whether treated patients really do better than those receiving no treatment. Now, one toxic treatment would only be compared to another toxic treatment!

One of the few hold-out trials which insisted on retaining a no-treatment arm was that of the West Midlands Cooperative Group.

Noticeably, like the Guy's-Manchester Trial before it, the West Midlands Trial also failed to show any significant benefit to adjuvant treatment, even in premenopausal women, the group for whom benefit was supposedly unequivocal (394). But it hardly seemed to matter. Adjuvant chemotherapy was on the map.

Too much adjuvant therapy?

"By the end of 1981," breast cancer activist Rose Kushner recalled, "I sensed that indiscriminate, automatic adjuvant chemotherapy was replacing the Halsted radical mastectomy as therapeutic overkill in the United States" (219). "The treatment of this tumor now has slipped from too much surgery to too much adjuvant therapy," Thomas Nealon, Jr., Professor of Surgery at New York University School of Medicine concluded at the ACS Science Writers' Seminar (281).

What really opened the floodgates were an urgent May, 1988 Clinical Alert from the National Cancer Institute, followed by four studies in the *New England Journal of Medicine* (123,124,238,247).

The Clinical Alert was a letter sent to thousands of practitioners across the U.S. urging them in no uncertain terms to start administering adjuvant chemotherapy to all breast cancer patients with negative axillary (armpit) nodes. The Alert bypassed the usual peer-review mechanisms that scientific findings are supposed to go through before being made public. The justification for this astonishing letter was the claim that 15 to 20 percent of these women would relapse during the first five years after just surgery or surgery plus radiation. The letter went on to state that if all node-negative women were treated "thousands of lives could be saved each year in the United States."

"This Clinical Alert sent shock waves through the oncology community and almost mandated that all women be treated simply because of the statement issued by the National Cancer Institute," Charles Simone, M.D. recalled (345). Under NCI's schema, he said, at least 80 percent of the women would be treated unnecessarily, the side effects would be incalculable, the cost would be monstrous, and there would be serious legal implications for the doctor.

"If a physician decided not to treat such a patient," he asked, "could that physician be held legally responsible?" (345)

In the following year, four studies came out in the *New England Journal* that appeared to lend credence to NCI's Clinical Alert. "These studies led to a dramatic increase in the use of chemotherapy for node-negative patients," wrote Austin and Hitchcock (26).

Bernard Fisher, leader of the NSABP, boldly declared, "There should be no vacillation whatsoever. Every patient should either go into a clinical trial or should be given the therapies" (306).

The articles purported to show major advantages for women with breast cancer through the use of adjuvant chemotherapy.

Oncologists examined various regimens. In one, women received a single course of CMF within 36 hours of breast surgery (238). In another, they received twelve four-week cycles of methotrexate + fluorouracil + leucovorin rescue within 30 days of their surgery (123). In the third, ER+ women received just tamoxifen (124). And finally, a group of women received six four-week cycles of the CMFP protocol (247). The controls received no treatment other than their initial surgery.

After four years, in each study there was a small to moderate difference in disease-free intervals. In the women who received a single course of CMF, for instance, 77 percent experienced a four-year disease-free interval compared to 74 percent in the control group. Those who received the most intensive treatment, CMFP, had an 84 percent disease-free interval compared to 69 percent in the controls (247).

However—and this would seem to be the important thing—in none of these studies was there any *actual survival* advantage. Once again, women were not really living any longer; they were simply having fewer "disease events" during the four-year period in question. This point was generally glossed over by boosters of chemotherapy.

90

In June, 1990, the NIH decided to hold a major conference on the treatment of early stage breast cancer. They assembled experts to come to some agreement on this disputed question. These experts were expected to provide doctors with guidelines on how to treat their breast cancer patients who had negative axillary nodes. But after days of deliberation, they were unable to issue a definitive statement and in effect dumped the decision back into the laps of the front-line doctors and their patients.

"All patients," they declared, "with node-negative breast cancer should be made aware of the benefits and risks of adjuvant systemic therapy, a thorough discussion of which should include the likely risk of recurrence without adjuvant therapy, the expected reduction in risk with adjuvant therapy, the toxic effects of therapy, and the impact of therapy on quality of life. Some degrees of improvement may be so small that the disadvantages of therapy outweigh them" (280).

After reviewing 10 randomized trials, they concluded that adjuvant systemic therapy did reduce the rate of recurrence by about one-third, but had no visible effect on improving the overall survival rate.

What do all the numbers mean?

Let us say that there 100 node-negative women who have been operated on for breast cancer. Their tumors were small and they have favorable histological types of cancer. Out of this group, 90 will not have a recurrence. They will be fine without any further treatment.

Of the ten who can be expected to experience a recurrence, three could probably benefit from adjuvant chemotherapy. Hence, toxic chemotherapy is given to 100 women in order to benefit three.

Studies have shown that about 70,000 U.S. women per year are diagnosed with breast cancer with negative axillary nodes. It has been estimated that 5,040 of these women could "benefit" in terms of disease-free intervals (again, with no proof of benefit in overall survival or lifespan). To achieve that goal for these 5,040 women, 64,960 other women have to be treated with toxic drugs. They cannot and will not derive *any* benefit from this treatment. They will have to suffer the side effects and the danger of death. And their cost (in 1989 dollars) would be about $340 million per year (252,345). And that is how "thousands of lives could be saved each year in the United States," NCI-style.

The Trialists' Study

In 1992, *The Lancet* published a huge "meta-analysis" of *all* the trials that had begun before 1985 on the treatment of early breast cancer with hormonal, cytotoxic, or immune therapy (108). Although the results have been interpreted as a boost for combination chemotherapy, when looked at closely, they are no more confirmatory than the above studies.

For 11,000 women looked at ten years after their participation in an RCT, these British "Trialists" seemed to show a 6.3 percent survival advantage for all such patients (51.3 percent vs. 45 percent). For node-negative women the advantage was *just 4 percent* (67.2 percent vs. 63.2 percent). For node positive women it was *less than 7 percent* (46.6 percent vs. 39.8 percent). This small difference led two researchers from Manitoba to write the *Lancet* that "no overall survival advantage has been seen so far" (336). If there is an advantage, it certainly has to be a small one in human terms.

The Trialists also found that for women under the age of 50, ablation (i.e., the removal or destruction) of the ovaries was "of comparable efficacy" to chemotherapy. This is an extremely important finding that has gotten little attention so far. It means that one relatively simple operation or a three-day radiological procedure can be substituted for months of risky drugs, with all their attendant side effects (308). Such surgery has been practiced since 1901 (30) and appears safe and moderately effective. Premenopausal women contemplating chemotherapy should certainly investigate this option.

The Trialists also found quite definitively that six months' of chemotherapy was as effective as twelve months. Women who are told they need eight or twelve full courses of treatment should also question their doctors on this point.

Quality of life issues

Adjuvant chemotherapy for breast cancer has been called "a biological experiment" whose "ultimate goal must be the improvement of the life of a woman suffering from early breast cancer" (394). Does adjuvant chemotherapy actually improve the lives of women?

It should hardly be surprising by now that no detailed records are kept on the side effects, obvious or subtle, of adjuvant chemotherapy. "There are no studies which have taken account of all these factors," said Dr. Alan Wilson (394). In fact, many oncologists seem disinterested in such mundane topics as quality of life or the costs to the patient. It has been found that when doctors are doing the recording, side effects are routinely underestimated (244).

"Most of the time, oncologists do not even see their patients during regular...appointments," complained activist Rose Kushner, shortly before her own death from breast cancer. "In the United States, baldness, nausea and vomiting, diarrhea, clogged veins, financial problems, broken marriages, disturbed children, loss of libido, loss of self-esteem, and body image are nurses' turf" (219). But "nurses don't publish studies of chemotherapy trials," Austin and Hitchcock added dryly (26).

Adjuvant treatment can be rough and can take its toll not just on the patient, but on friends and family. In the NSABP trial, for two years the patients had to have blood tests every three weeks and physical examinations every month and a half for two years (142). Usually, someone had to help them get to the appointment—and back.

Chemotherapy is sometimes continued even when there are severe side effects. In three NSABP protocols there was serious (grade II) blood toxicity in 290 instances. Yet in 157 cases chemotherapy was continued despite the fact that the protocol itself demanded that this severe a degree of toxicity results in cessation of treatment (143).

The use of such combination chemotherapy "demands a high degree of expertise." Medical oncologists have been called "rare birds" in the United Kingdom, as they are in most of the world. One wonders about the social cost of training and maintaining a large cadre of subspecialists to perform such marginally successful procedures.

Side effects

A few patients claim that adjuvant chemotherapy is like a "day at the beach" (224). But the vast majority of patients suffer side effects during such treatment. A 1994 survey found that "patients reported a mean of 3.2 to 4.9 side effects at each point in time" (157). Most common were fatigue, nausea, anorexia, taste changes, and headache.

In the Milan trial, 98 percent of the patients had some degree of toxicity. In another study, 52 patients were randomized to either the standard Milan CMF protocol or to a lower-dose CMF regimen. Of those receiving the standard dose, 78 percent suffered nausea and vomiting, compared to "only" 14 percent in the low-dose category. Incidence of hair loss so severe that it required wearing a wig ranged from 4 percent in Milan to 36 percent in Glasgow (393).

Dr. Bonadonna says that those who refuse to complete his treatment are not really being poisoned by his drugs, but are just "psychologically disturbed" by the very idea of therapy. To me, this sounds like a case of blaming the victim (42).

Even the vice president of the ACS, John Laszlo, M.D., has said that about a quarter of long-term chemotherapy patients become "conditioned" to experience symptoms even in the absence of the actual drugs themselves. In his book, *Understanding Cancer*, he wrote:

"We have seen patients drive into the hospital parking lot and promptly begin to vomit, or vomit when they smell the alcohol sponge used to clean off the arm prior to chemotherapy or even vomit when they see the nurse who administers the chemotherapy—even if that person is encountered out of uniform in a supermarket or elsewhere away from the hospital" (225).

But in a controlled trial, it was 59 percent of patients—not one quarter, as Laszlo suggests—who vomited merely by anticipating the full CMF treatment (393).

Long-term problems

In addition, there can be long-term problems. Some oncologists claim that the patient's standard blood profile springs back to normal after a few months. But blood damage can also be subtle and long-lasting.

There is, for instance, a phenomenon called late bone marrow failure. "This morbidity to stem cells" (i.e., progenitor cells of the blood-making system) "is not initially reflected by peripheral blood counts...," two British authors wrote. "However, repeated drug administration causes cumulative toxicity..." (199). Other serious side effects:

• "Weight gain is a common side effect that may decrease quality of life and potentially threaten survival," wrote scientists at Duke University (94). There is no explanation for why this occurs.

• Seven percent of women receiving chemotherapy for breast cancer experienced blood clots, compared to no such clots in controls (16).

• The CMF protocol, when started within 36 hours of mastectomy, has been responsible for at least four deaths attributed to a potentiation of the drug methotrexate by the nitrous oxide anesthetic (237).

• Other patients have succumbed to "toxic deaths" in the course of these trials (142,251). According to the EORTC, "*It appears that the mortality rate of regimens containing methotrexate is about one percent*" (394). Methotrexate is the "M" in the common "CMF" protocol.

The bottom line

The bottom line is that after twenty years, it is still unclear if adjuvant chemotherapy in premenopausal women actually cures a greater proportion of patients than good supportive care alone, or only postpones relapses and death. "As long as this question cannot be answered," said Abel, "it remains open whether adjuvant chemotherapy reduces breast cancer mortality by a measurable amount" (3).

The treatment of advanced breast cancer

Chemotherapy, usually in combinations, is also widely used in the treatment of metastasized breast disease. In fact, over two dozen drugs have been approved for this use. Our discussion of this topic will be shorter and simpler. There is no evidence that chemotherapy can cure people with advanced breast disease.

Nonetheless, it is widely believed that even if chemotherapy does not actually cure such cancers, it is worth administering because it extends life or improves life quality. But is this really the case?

The Cooper Regimen

In the 1970s and '80s, there was a great deal of excitement over a combination of five drugs and hormones called the "Cooper regimen" (CMFVP). It was said that this brought about a high rate of responses. However, despite the publicity, these claims were never adequately proven (69). Although this regimen still has its adherents, according to Dr. DeVita's textbook it is now used less frequently "because of severe myelosuppression and neurotoxicity without clear-cut evidence of a superior long-term benefit" (97). In fact, a Swiss study suggested that in some cases a "more aggressive simultaneous hormone-chemo-therapy" program resulted in "significantly worse survival" than that seen in patients who took drugs one by one (64).

Although there have been over 230 trials on advanced breast cancer alone (241), there is still no direct evidence that chemotherapy actually prolongs survival. A German Consensus Development Conference concluded that "there may be patient subgroups in which chemotherapy prolongs survival. However, at present, these groups cannot be defined precisely" (80).

The reason for this lack of precision is that, once again, almost all studies regard "response rates" as the main end point of a clinical trial. However, as is stated in the European (EORTC) review, response rates are "of limited value when assessing overall therapeutic benefit in an incurable disease like advanced breast cancer" (241). There are no controlled studies in advanced breast cancer that compare chemotherapy to untreated controls. Nor are there any randomized comparisons of patients given immediate vs. deferred chemotherapy.

Hormones work better

There have, however, been a number of large and well-documented studies that compared hormonal agents either before or alongside chemotherapy in older women who had stage IV breast cancer. The surprising result, however, was that patients actually did better when given hormonal therapy *alone* than when it was given in combination with chemotherapy. Thus, starting with hormonal therapy "is not only significantly less toxic but induced a slightly longer survival" time than the CMF regimen, according to a report in the *Annals of Internal Medicine* in 1986 (362).

Combination superior?

Although it is current dogma that combinations of agents work better than single agents, actual results have not supported this conclusion, regardless of the combination employed. In fact, five studies actually showed a *decreased* response rate with combinations—women died sooner. Even those studies that claimed an increased response *rate*, did not show any corresponding increase in *duration* of that response or in actual survival.

Single agent vs. single agent

Some studies have compared one single agent vs. another. It didn't make much difference. Although minor variations in response rates were observed, "none of these was significant and no survival differences were seen" (241).

Combinations on different schedules

There have also been over 30 randomized studies in which the same combination of drugs was administered, but in differing intensities, routes of administration or time of administration. In some, the survival data wasn't even recorded! In others, the number of women was too small to yield meaningful results (3).

Maximal dose better?

Was a more intensive regimen better than a milder one? In one study, a small survival advantage was in fact seen in women receiving high doses of CMF compared to those receiving lower doses. This is often used to justify more aggressive treatment. But the advantage amounted to *less than three months of increased life* (15.6 vs. 12.8 months median survival) (359). Upon closer analysis, it turned out there were major differences in the selection criteria of the two groups and that once these were adjusted for the survival differences became statistically non-significant (3). We can conclude that there is no adequate proof of significant survival differences in favor of more intensive regimens (173,174,307). Abel calls this "amazing" in the light of all the studies done (3).

The sober judgment of a group of German oncologists thus seems inescapable: "[T]he widespread opinion that, in order to achieve optimal effect, chemotherapy for metastasized breast cancer has to be given in maximal dose approaching the verge of tolerance is erroneous, especially in routine use: while toxic side-effects caused by elevated doses considerably increase, a significant improvement in response rates or survival is not demonstrable" (307).

Shrinkages and survival

It is in breast cancer that we most often hear the claim that tumor shrinkages result in improved survival. One group of scientists has claimed that after studying 50 published trials of chemotherapy in advanced breast cancer, they found that "in 73 percent of comparisons the group with the higher response rate also demonstrated the longer median survival" (8). However, they then admitted that "trials rarely demonstrate a statistically significant survival advantage," undercutting their own thesis. If a study is not statistically significant it is virtually meaningless as proof.

In 1990, British scientists concluded: "Recent years have seen the introduction of therapies capable of shrinking disease volume although the concept of a cure still remains remote....[M]any of these treatments are unpleasant and the burden they force the patient to bear may not be compensated by the reduction in tumor size" (29).

After surveying the various randomized studies the European (EORTC) reviewers concluded that *"a consistent and striking feature is the lack of correlation between higher response rates and prolonged survival"* (241) (emphasis added).

Survival data

Data showing an historical increase in survival for some groups of patients is sometimes used to "prove" that treatment is working. For example, three-year survival increased 11 percent in Norway in the early 1970s, just around the time that combination chemotherapy came into use. At one Texas clinic, it was found that patients with liver metastases were living 14 months, while in an earlier decade they only survived 5 months (64).

Grandiose conclusions are sometimes drawn from such small studies. By contrast, a major study that contrasted results drawn from 100 hospitals found that both three- and five-year survival rates had actually *deteriorated* between the 1950s and the 1960s (274). Other studies from the 1980s also revealed no improvement in survival statistics after the introduction of combination chemotherapy (206,309,310,366). In fact, "most retrospective studies have failed to show that the survival of patients with advanced breast cancer has changed very much over the past 20 to 30 years" (173).

Our conclusion is the same as that of two German scientists who wrote: "We think that from the ethical point of view it seems problematic to apply aggressive chemotherapy programs to patients with metastatic disease since no significant therapeutic effect in terms of prolongation of life span can be assumed" (299).

Bone marrow transplantation

At this writing, there is special interest in the topic of bone marrow transplantation (BMT) with high-dose chemotherapy for breast cancer. An extraordinary situation has developed in which women with advanced breast cancer are demanding this treatment, moving heaven and earth to obtain it, while the medical establishment admits it does not have any idea whether it is any better than conventional treatment. In 1994, at least 1,000 women in the U.S. received BMT outside the context of clinical trials (211).

The NCI has currently scheduled three high-priority clinical trials to compare BMT with conventional chemotherapy. But, as indicated, it is having trouble getting cancer patients to enroll in the trial, because the word is out on the ineffectiveness of standard chemotherapy. "Scientists say they are worried that without proper studies no one will ever know whether the new treatment is actually better," according to the *New York Times* (211).

Patients should know that BMT is a "grueling, risky and expensive" treatment. Its use has raised major economic conflicts, since "doctors and hospitals stand to gain if an expensive new treatment is approved" while "insurance companies benefit if the old, cheaper treatment remains standard." Meanwhile, "researchers' careers are staked on the completion of clinical studies" (211).

While most insurance companies initially refused to pay for this treatment, "after several lawsuits, many insurance companies changed their policies and some states passed laws mandating coverage."

What does the record actually show on the effectiveness of BMTs? Not much. The PDQ system of NCI distributes a 20,000-word statement on breast cancer that contains but a single paragraph on BMTs (57). According to this statement, "for metastatic disease, high-dose chemotherapy with autologous bone marrow transplantation (ABMT) has been associated with a high response rate, although responses are generally not of long duration" (24,209).

Colon and rectum

The colon is the large intestine. Including the rectum, it forms the last seven feet or so of the human digestive tract. Because of the similarities between colon and rectal cancer, these are sometimes considered as a single category, colorectal cancer.

In 1995, there will be an estimated 138,200 new cases in the U.S., 100,000 of the colon and 38,200 of the rectum. There will be an estimated 55,300 deaths, 47,500 from colon, 7,800 from rectal cancer (11).

The death rate for males with colon and rectal cancer varies around the world from a mere 2.7 in Ecuador to a high of 30.7 per 100,000 in the former Czechoslovakia—a differential of over 10 times. Other countries with high rates are Hungary, New Zealand, Ireland, Denmark, Germany and Austria (10). In the United States the rate is approximately in the middle, with 16.7 deaths per 100,000 people.

Diet and life style are presumed to be very important in its causation: countries with high rates tend to be those with a high intake of saturated fats from meat. Those with low rates tend to be those where people eat lots of fiber-containing grains, legumes, and vegetables (e.g., rice and beans), and small amounts of protein, mainly in the form of chicken and fish.

Curable through surgery

In its early stages, localized colon cancer is considered curable through surgery. Most if not all colon cancers are now believed to derive from premalignant polyps in the intestinal tract. Some people have a hereditary tendency to form polyps, and genetic tests for family susceptibility are being developed. Through the use of early diagnosis and surgery, cure rates for this type of cancer may improve in the future.

In colon cancer, the staging system is different than in most other cancers. Instead of the TNM system, or the roman numeral subgroups, staging is usually based on a system devised by the British pathologist, Cuthbert E. Dukes (1890-1977). Dukes' A is essentially the equivalent of stage I, Dukes' B1 and Dukes' B2 of stage II, Dukes' C1 and Dukes' C2 of stage III, and Dukes' D of stage IV.

Once the disease has begun to spread, long-term survival rates plummet. The five-year survival in Dukes' D is only 5 percent, but is said to be 20 percent if liver metastases can be surgically removed.

In stages Dukes' A, B and C, the primary treatment of choice is surgery. In Dukes' D, where the cancer has already spread to distant sites, surgery is sometimes used palliatively, but the disease is considered virtually incurable by conventional means.

Chemotherapy is becoming more common in its treatment:

Treatment of Colon Cancer in U.S. Hospitals

Year	Surgery & Chemo	Surg. Rad. & Chemo	Chemo
1985/86	6.8	1.4	1.4
1991	18.7	1.9	2.1

Treatment of Rectal Cancer in U.S. Hospitals

Year	Surgery & Chemo	Surg. Rad. & Chem	Chemo
1985/86	3.1	5.3	0.9
1991	7.6	19.2	1.4

Thus, almost a quarter of all colon cancer patients received in-hospital chemotherapy, almost always following surgery, while nearly 30 percent of all rectal cancer patients received it. Extrapolating from the above statistics, we can estimate that at least 36,000 Americans will receive in-hospital chemotherapy for colorectal cancer in 1995.

Dukes' B

In Dukes' B colon cancer, five-year survival rates are 70 to 80 percent and "nearly half of the deaths are due to causes other than cancer."

For this reason, even the NCI says that adjuvant chemotherapy should not only *not* be routinely recommended but "should be offered ...only in the context of a clinical trial" (275).

Duke's C (regionally spread) colon cancer

The big news in the treatment of Dukes' C colon cancer has been the claim that patients given a combination of two agents, fluorouracil (5-FU) and levamisole after surgery, have increased disease-free as well as absolute survival compared to those who have had surgery alone.

Enthusiasm for 5-FU and levamisole probably accounts for the greatly increased use of chemotherapy seen in the above NCDB figures. As that report puts it, "Treatment trends are beginning to show the effects of clinical trial data, as evidenced by the use of multi-modality therapy for certain stages of colon and rectal cancer" (355).

In fact, 5-FU alone had been a common treatment for advanced colorectal cancer for many years. However, "many early trials of adjuvant chemotherapy failed to show a significant improvement in either overall or disease-free survival for patients receiving treatment...," according to the government's PDQ report (275).

Any overall survival benefit "if it indeed exists, would likely be small: the effect of prolonged fluorouracil-containing chemotherapy results in a five-year survival benefit of less than 5 percent" (275).

However, the picture changed entirely in 1990 when Charles Moertel, M.D. of the Mayo Clinic, Rochester, MN, published a study on the adjuvant use of 5-FU and levamisole, started within five weeks of surgery, in the treatment of stage Dukes' C colon cancer (265). This report generated headlines that made it seem as if the cure for colon cancer was at hand.

Levamisole was and is a standard de-worming agent for sheep and other animals. Since the early 1970s it has also been known to have immune system-modulating effects as well. In the abovementioned Mayo Clinic study, a combination of these two agents was compared to the use of levamisole alone, as well as to a control group that received no adjuvant treatment at all.

Results of Mayo study

This study purported to show a 41 percent decrease in the rate of recurrence and, more importantly, a 33 percent decrease in the death rate over doing nothing after surgery. Although technically speaking, this was not a study of chemotherapy *per se*, but of cytotoxic chemotherapy plus a kind of immunotherapy, we will consider it here.

This was a large, apparently well-controlled study, headed by a renowned chemotherapist at a prestigious center. It changed the treatment of colorectal cancer, and infused new hope into oncology as a whole. In May 1990, this treatment was officially recommended by an NIH Consensus Conference on Colon Cancer.

Its results have essentially been duplicated by an even larger multi-center study, with the participation of some of the largest cooperative groups in the country. This second study enrolled 1,296 patients, of whom 929 were in stage C (266). At three years, the report claimed to see overall survival of 71 percent in the adjuvant treatment group vs. 55 percent in the surgery group. This is a survival advantage of 33 percent. And at five years, the Mayo scientists said, the same "one-third reduction in cancer mortality can still be demonstrated" (75).

If these results hold up, then 5-FU and levamisole would certainly seem to be a rational treatment for stage C colon cancer. However, there seems to be some hedging over their significance. Thus, while NCI still upholds the idea that a "significant improvement in disease-free survival was observed," it now adds that "overall survival benefits were of borderline statistical significance" (275).

NCI's recommendation for Dukes' C seems rather weak: "Patients should be considered for adjuvant therapy with 5-FU and levamisole, or with one of the other regimens now being studied in clinical trials." And, in fact, oncologists are now saying that the main significance of the Mayo study was the impetus it gave for further clinical trials (75).

Those contemplating the 5-FU and levamisole treatment for Dukes' C colon cancer should consider the following facts:

Short-term toxicity

Despite a general consensus that side effects are "mild and reversible" (75), levamisole alone can sometimes have significant toxicity. Its most serious side effect is *granulocytopenia*, a deficiency of the most common kind of white blood cell. In 1994, a study also found a possible inhibition of liver function when 5-FU and levamisole were given at the same time as the common drug, warfarin (333,401). It is believed to have caused some cases of encephalitis in a large Chinese study of peasants who had been given this medication as a treatment for intestinal worms (403). It can also cause nausea, abdominal pain, vomiting, diarrhea, a metallic or altered taste, fatigue, arthralgias, flu-like symptoms, tremors, agitation, insomnia, hyper-alertness, dizziness, headache, and confusion (75,272). Some immunotherapy!

Long-term toxicity

Levamisole alone was also given at the Harbor–UCLA Hospital in Torrance, CA as an adjuvant treatment for colon cancer, starting in 1975. A recent analysis of the long-term outcome in those patients raised *the disturbing possibility that levamisole is a long-term poison.*

When it was given alone as an adjuvant after surgery it seriously decreased the survival time of patients with both Dukes' B and C colorectal cancer. In a 1994 paper, Rowan Chlebowski, M.D., Ph.D., and colleagues showed that while *five-year* survival was comparable for those receiving either levamisole or a placebo (sugar pill), "subsequent survival favored placebo over levamisole" (70).

Overall survival was 68 percent in the placebo group but only 38 percent in the levamisole-treatment group! In other words, in the long run, the use of levamisole greatly *decreased* survival in these cancer patients compared to doing nothing. Dr. Chlebowski and his colleagues concluded that any long-term use of levamisole and 5-FU should be carefully examined, and that "future trials" using levamisole "should proceed cautiously" (70).

For some, this finding was not surprising, for in a large clinical trial in 1981, levamisole alone seemed to adversely affect both the response rate and the survival of a different kind of malignancy (i.e., non-small-cell lung cancer) (93).

No analogous results

It is puzzling that levamisole has not shown comparable results as an adjuvant treatment for any other kind of cancer. A trial in malignant melanoma showed no difference between the treatment and the control groups (352). Nor does it even work in either Dukes' B or Dukes' D colon cancer—certainly an odd circumstance.

No known mechanism of action

Beyond the rather vague term "immunostimulant," no actual mechanism of action has yet been proposed for the alleged anticancer effects of levamisole. In fact, Dr. Moertel of the Mayo Clinic himself noted that "it is difficult to explain why this empirically conceived drug combination is effective" (265).

No effect on statistics

The NCDB figures show that the stepped up use of chemotherapy in colon cancer has not yet had any effect on survival statistics. "Overall survival for colon cancer is not different from what has been reported in the past and in other data bases," the authors said in 1994. "Reports that allude to recently improved survival in all patients with large-bowel cancer are not yet documentable by the NCDB" (355).

Excessive cost

The Mayo Clinic's Dr. Moertel himself became an outspoken crusader against the giant manufacturer of levamisole, Johnson & Johnson (J&J). He pointed out that as a de-wormer, levamisole cost about $1 per year. But as soon as it was accepted for human use—mainly as a result of his own efforts—J&J upped the price to $1,200 per year (*Los Angeles Times*, 9/11/93).

Conclusions

In conclusion then, it would be odd if one drug that does not increase survival (5-FU), added to another which actually *decreases* survival (levamisole), together prolonged peoples' lives. Certainly, stranger things have happened, but caution is advised both in interpreting the data and in taking this treatment.

Dukes' D (stage IV)

Overall, about 30 to 40 percent of patients with colorectal cancer fall into this category upon diagnosis. Essentially, says NCI, "there is no standard chemotherapy for patients with widespread metastatic disease"(275). Simply put, nothing conventional really works.

The "response rate" with 5-FU or 5-FU-containing combinations is said to be up to 20 percent. By adding leucovorin rescue factor, a drug that facilitates higher doses of cytotoxic agents, the response rate can be bumped up somewhat. One study claimed a 48 percent response rate, but this was probably a flawed result, since it "was obtained by omitting five patients who died during the first course" of treatment. It was also "probably biased since the study was broken off when differences were observed between the treatments" (3).

Complete remissions are rare and in any case do not correlate with increased survival. In fact, there is no evidence that survival is actually improved by chemotherapy.

An early study seemed to show promising survival benefits for a technique called portal-vein infusion (361). Overall, however, a number of large trials have now failed to demonstrate a significant benefit for such treatment in the reduction of liver recurrences, according to the PDQ (275).

Lung

Lung cancer is the leading cause of cancer deaths in the United States for both men and women. There will be an estimated 169,900 new U.S. cases in 1995, with 157,400 deaths (11).

The death rate for lung cancer in men ranges from a low of 6.9 per 100,000 in Ecuador to 76.4 per 100,000 in Hungary. Other countries with high rates include Czechoslovakia, Scotland, Netherlands, and Poland. Among women, the U.S. is the second highest country, after Scotland, with 24.7 per 100,000. The lowest rate for women is found in Ecuador, with a remarkably low 2.8 per 100,000 (10).

Lung cancer is one of the major types of cancer for which the death rate among women is rising dramatically, presumably due to increased smoking. It is categorized into two main varieties, small-cell (SCLC) and non-small-cell lung cancer (NSCLC). Each of these comes in several subtypes as well, and will be considered separately.

Small-cell lung cancer

Small-cell lung cancer is of particular interest because it is one of the very few forms of carcinoma for which chemotherapy has in fact been *proven to have a positive effect on survival*. But this effect is measured in terms *of weeks or months*, not years.

The varieties of SCLC include oat cell, intermediate, and combined types. SCLC accounts for about 20 percent of all newly diagnosed lung cancer cases. It tends to metastasize readily and grow rapidly. It therefore carries a poor prognosis. SCLC is generally classified into limited or extensive types, rather than by the typical

TNM classifications.

It is sometimes claimed that chemotherapy is quite effective in SCLC. "The outlook for those with tumors of small-cell origin has been dramatically improved by chemotherapy," said Dr. Elaine M. Rankin (314). Dr. Daniel Ihde, until 1994 deputy director of the NCI, has written in a similar vein:

"Introduction of effective combination chemotherapy with or without chest irradiation into the management of SCLC had led to four- to five-fold improvement in median survival compared with survival of untreated patients and a small fraction of patients in whom the tumor is permanently eradicated" (396).

What he doesn't say is that the median survival using combinations of chemotherapy and radiation has rarely if ever been shown to be increased by more than a few months (245).

Nonetheless, the treatment of SCLC is held up as a paradigm to be followed in the treatment of other cancers. Again according to Dr. Ihde, SCLC is said to be "similar to other cancers in which chemotherapy yields major improvement in survival and some cures..." (395). If we restrict ourselves to a discussion of randomized controlled studies, however, the record in no way supports such optimistic projections.

SCLC was and remains a generally fatal disease, in which chemotherapy has definite but limited success. If the cancer has spread outside of the lung, the definition of *extensive disease*, it will almost certainly cause the death of the conventionally treated patient.

According to the U.S. government's SEER data, five-year relative survival for SCLC is 5 percent, but only 1.6 percent in cases with distant spread. More than half the cases already have such distant spread when they are diagnosed (323). And there is no standard test for use in early diagnosis, and so many patients are discovered in the later stages.

The oncologist who did the European (EORTC) review has said that SCLC is "a difficult tumor in which to achieve effective long-term survival" despite its sensitivity to both radio- and chemotherapy (245).

Placebo-controlled studies

Few studies have actually compared survival with drugs and/ or radiotherapy vs. placebo. One such study, published in 1969, compared 57 patients who received cyclophosphamide with 87 who received just placebo (154). Median survival time was 16 weeks in the treatment group and 6 weeks in the placebo group. (Median survival means that half the group lived longer, half shorter than the mean number.) Technically, therefore, in the manner of NCI's Dr. Ihde, one could truthfully say that treatment tripled survival time, although this tripling represented *an actual survival gain of just 10 weeks.*

In 1982, doctors gave one group placebo, while two similar groups got either ifosfamide or ifosfamide + CCNU (217). The placebo group had a median survival of 42 days, while the chemotherapy groups lived between 107 to 110 days. Again, chemotherapy nearly tripled their median survival time, this time for *a net gain of about two months.*

Many people would say that a few months are better than nothing. But the control group had advantages in quality of life because of their freedom from side effects. Ifosfamide is a notoriously toxic drug (120,203). For some, the combination caused destruction of white blood cells; hair loss; severe nausea and vomiting; and hemorrhagic cystitis, whose symptoms range from blood in the urine to full-scale bleeding that may require the intervention of a urologist. (Mesna is usually given with ifosfamide as a bladder-protecting agent.)

Comparative studies

There are at least six comparative studies of various drugs for SCLC (62,77,110,164,165,234) and all of them show basically the same thing: a few months' survival benefit to the patient, with greater toxicity the more intensive and complex the drug treatment becomes.

Median survival in such studies ranged as high as 7.6 months (227 days) in one study from the Finsen Institute in Copenhagen, although this was scaled back to 5.8 months (176 days) in a larger study at the same center (164,165).

A 1977 study at NCI (77) created excitement with a claim of 10.5 months median survival compared to just 5.0 months in the standard-dose group. But a larger study saw no difference in survival (57). There was, however, "a considerable incidence of toxicity in the group treated with high-intensity induction chemotherapy" (245).

Salvage therapy

Chemotherapy is often given after a relapse in so-called salvage therapy. But even NCI's Dr. Ihde admits that "chemotherapy infrequently yields objective tumor responses in patients with relapsed SCLC; it is almost never of benefit in patients whose tumor progresses while the initial chemotherapy program is being administered" (395).

Compared to radiation

A 1975 trial compared chemotherapy with hemibody (half-body) irradiation. The median survival time with radiation was 218 days, compared to just 87 days for those receiving a combination of four drugs.

This advantage held true for the overall group as well as for each age group considered separately. And although radiation is certainly not free of side effects, chemotherapy caused more effects and achieved less palliation than radiation (222). SCLC patients who are considering chemotherapy might want to seek a second opinion from a qualified radiation oncologist.

Conclusions

• In SCLC, there *is* evidence of increased survival using chemotherapy. But this survival benefit is of only a few months' duration and seems to be equalled or excelled by radiation therapy.
• Combination chemotherapy has not been proven to be significantly better than single-agent treatment.
• The side effects of drugs, especially high-dose, multi-drug regimens, can be punishing. In some studies, up to two-thirds of patients had life-threatening toxicity (234) and some died "toxic deaths" from the treatment itself (258).

Non-small-cell lung

Non-small-cell lung cancer (NSCLC) is statistically far more common than SCLC, accounting for about 75 to 80 percent of all cases of lung cancers in industrial countries. There are three different types of NSCLC: squamous cell, large cell, and adenocarcinomas. Squamous cell carcinoma is the most common but, for reasons unknown, the incidence of adenocarcinoma is increasing rapidly.

Squamous cell lung cancer is most closely linked to smoking and is therefore generally preventable (by smoking cessation). While some people appear to have been cured by surgery, the five-year survival rate for NSCLC remains only ten percent. The conventional treatment of choice is surgery and/or radiation. Chemotherapy is supposed to be reserved for patients with extensive or metastatic disease (314). In stage IV, when NSCLC has already spread to distant sites, five-year survival is 1.6 percent (323).

Yet, ironically, NSCLC is another one of those cancers for which there is some evidence, albeit slender, that chemotherapy actually extends life. It therefore bears close scrutiny.

As an adjuvant

First of all, chemotherapy has been tried as an adjuvant treatment after surgery—similar to the way it is widely used in breast cancer. The hope was that the drugs would knock out the putative micrometastases that led to recurrences after surgery. But the results in general have "failed to demonstrate any advantage for adjuvant chemotherapy for resectable lung cancer" (314).

In the first study (58), in fact, as the EORTC's Dr. Rankin stated:

"There was a higher incidence of recurrence and death in the cyclophosphamide-treated group, raising the interesting point that the cyclophosphamide may have adversely affected the ability of the host to eradicate small tumor deposits" (314).

In a five-year study, the Veterans Administration Surgical Adjuvant Group failed to show any advantage to chemotherapy. In another study, survival at three years was slightly higher—in the control group. Finally, in a fourth study, there was no difference at 11 months. Rankin adds, "It is noteworthy that life-threatening thrombocytopenia [a kind of white blood cell destruction, ed.] occurred in 5 of the 36 patients treated with CCNU."

The conclusion on adjuvant use is simple: "The currently available chemotherapy drugs used alone or in combination do not have sufficient activity against tumors to justify their use in the adjuvant setting" (314).

Placebo-controlled studies

There have been several randomized comparisons of chemotherapy vs. placebo. In each trial, patients who received the drugs did live somewhat longer than the placebo controls (339). However, in only two did the difference reach statistical significance.

A small study claiming statistically significant survival was published in 1982 (83). The placebo group survived 8.5 weeks. Those receiving a regimen called MACC (methotrexate + doxorubicin + cyclophosphamide + lomustine) survived 30.5 weeks, *for a total gain of about five months.*

However, in another study using a combination of drugs on ambulatory patients, survival was 10 weeks in those receiving the combination but double that—20 weeks—in those receiving just one drug, cyclophosphamide alone.

"The severe toxicity of the combination probably contributed to its adverse influence on survival," the EORTC reviewer, Dr. Elaine M. Rankin, quietly remarked. And, she added, no regimen of standard drugs "clearly demonstrated a survival advantage for patients with non-small-cell lung cancer" (314).

Comparing agents

Half a dozen studies have showed no difference between one agent and another (e.g., 116). In some tests, a slight difference of a few weeks were seen between different agents, but with great toxicity in some patients (92,294).

Adding cisplatin

In the 1980s, many hopes were stirred by the addition of the new drug cisplatin to existing regimens, following the proven utility of this agent in the treatment of relatively rare testicular cancers. And in NSCLC cisplatin will indeed bring about temporary tumor shrinkages in many patients. One study also showed some increased survival of patients with the addition of platinol to a complex, multi-drug formula (132). Patients in the "standard" drug group had a median survival of 22.6 weeks, while those who also got the cisplatin-containing regimen lived 34.9 weeks — *a gain of about three months,* but enough to qualify for statistical significance according to the rules of the game.

But cisplatin has notorious toxicities. It is one of the five worst drugs for causing nausea and vomiting (232). It can damage the kidneys and ears and even permanently destroy one's hearing (143). Its effects on the bone marrow can lead to life-threatening infections, contributing to a higher incidence of "toxic deaths" in the platinol group (132).

With radiation

In addition, there have also been at least ten studies comparing combination chemotherapy plus radiation therapy to radiation therapy alone. "All of these studies failed to show any survival advantage of the combination," Abel summarizes (3). In another study, scientists added the chemotherapy regimen known as CAP (cyclophosphamide + doxorubicin + cisplatin) to radiation therapy. Their purpose was to improve the results when the tumors had been incompletely removed by surgery and were locally advanced. At one year, there was a slight advantage for the chemotherapy group, but this advantage disappeared after 30 months of follow-up (240).

Wait and see

It is an important point that *the greatest single predictor of survival in NSCLC is the patient's performance status.* It is therefore logical to compare the immediate use of chemotherapy with a more conservative, wait-and-see approach. In this latter approach, patients are only treated when and if they begin to physically deteriorate.

This was tried in two studies. In the first, doctors saw no difference in survival time between the two approaches; in the second study there was actually a survival advantage in putting off the drug treatment (222). And interestingly, 30 of the 51 patients in the group that did not immediately receive chemotherapy never had it prescribed for them before their deaths.

Scientists have also tried to find some difference between high-dose and low-dose regimens of chemotherapy. They compared immediate aggressive combination of cyclophosphamide + doxorubicin + methotrexate + procarbazine (CAMP) to a mild initial therapy (low-dose lomustine). There were no differences between the two groups, either in survival or quality of life (220). Even some partisans of chemotherapy concede that there is no need to immediately begin chemotherapy for this kind of cancer: "Therapy can be started when symptoms become worse or when the tumor becomes larger" (153).

Conclusions

There may be weak indications for a life-prolonging effect of cisplatin-containing combinations. However, these effects are quite small, and are purchased at a high cost in toxicity. People have died a "toxic death" in the course of such trials. "Despite the best efforts of surgeons, radiotherapists, and medical oncologists, the treatment of non-small-cell lung cancer is disheartening," said Dr. Rankin. "There is plenty of scope for improvement" (314). According to another doctor, "There has been no improvement in the survival rate in decades, which is a reflection of both the lack of a satisfactory screening test... and, up to the present time, the lack of truly effective treatment with clear survival benefit" (143).

Better left unsaid?

Writing in the professional journal *Chest* in 1991, oncologist Charles Haskell concluded that "the quantitative impact of chemotherapy on survival is minuscule." He recalled that there had been six RCTs that actually compared chemotherapy to best supportive care alone as the initial treatment. The use of chemotherapy resulted in a survival advantage of 1.1 months," he said. If one added cisplatin, the survival advantage climbed to 2.3 months. However, this is achieved at the cost of great expense and such side effects as "deafness, loss of taste, renal dysfunction, neuropathy, nausea, vomiting, bone marrow suppression, and the risk of toxic death" (170).

Why isn't this better known? You might think Dr. Haskell would want to shout such facts from the rooftops to save patients from having to undergo unnecessary treatments. Yet in a *Los Angeles Times* letter, he himself attacked Dr. Martin Shapiro for pointing out exactly such facts to the general public.

"Although much of what Shapiro says about the use of chemothera-py is technically true," said Dr. Haskell, "it is the 'truth' of the college sophomore who can be characterized as 'idea rich, but experience poor.' It is the 'truth' of a physician who appears to have forgotten the importance of hope in fighting life-threatening illness. It is the 'truth' of one who is ignorant of the stories of individual patients who have enjoyed prolonged survival after chemotherapy.

"It is a 'truth'," he concluded, "that would have been better left unsaid" (169).

Ovarian cancer

The highest rates of ovarian cancer are found in industrialized coun-tries, with the exception of Japan, which for reasons unknown has rates among the lowest in the world. In the U.S., ovarian cancer is the fourth most common malignancy in women and the most common fatal gyne-cological cancer. There will be an estimated 26,600 new U.S. cases in 1995, with 14,500 deaths (11).

Ovarian cancer is particularly difficult to treat, because although there is a relatively high long-term remission rate in early-stage disease, women usually have widespread disease by the time it is dis-covered. Symptoms are often vague and nonspecific and the necessity of doing an operation called a laparotomy for diagnosis may lead to fur-ther delays. Primarily for those reasons, the death rate from this type of cancer equals that for all other gynecological cancers combined.

Chemotherapy is used on nearly 60 percent of in-hospital patients, along with surgery and/or radiation, although there has been little increase in usage between 1985-86 and 1991.

Treatment of Ovarian Cancer in U.S. Hospitals

Year	Surg. & Chemo	Surg. Rad. & Chemo	Chemo
1985/86	44.9	1.7	11.4
1991	46.9	1.0	9.0

Figuring on the basis of 26,600 new U.S. cases in 1995, we can see that over 15,000 of them will receive in-hospital chemotherapy each year. This figure is probably higher today, since the introduction of new drugs after the NCDB survey was conducted.

Surgery is still the primary treatment for ovarian cancer. It is consid-ered extremely important to remove as much as possible of residual tumor, and to achieve a complete remission, if possible, through radia-tion and/or chemotherapy. "The oncologic gospel," said Dr. Maurice

L. Slevin, "is that small is beautiful" (347).

Ovarian cancer is one of the few types of carcinoma for which chemotherapy *does appear to significantly prolong life*. Unlike in lung cancer, *the increase may be a year or more*. However, despite the likelihood that this is so, it is surprising to find that even here there is a lack of good direct evidence for this benefit.

Chemotherapy is generally begun one to two weeks after surgery. Patients frequently receive, intravenously, one of the platinum-containing drugs, cisplatin or carboplatin, plus cyclophosphamide. They receive this every three to four weeks for at least six cycles.

Combinations vs. Single Drugs

Once again, we find that the trend towards complicated multi-drug regimens, which require a more intensive involvement by oncologists, is not necessarily more effective than single agents.

Single drugs can provide symptomatic relief "at the cost of very little toxicity," said the EORTC's Dr. Slevin. Again we hear the old complaint: that "more intensive chemotherapy gives greater response rates, but there is no prolongation of survival in most patients" (347). As noted, survivors in the most advanced cases, so-called FIGO stage IV, are rare. Therefore, it makes little sense to give them high-dose toxic chemotherapy.

Many chemotherapists believe their main goal should be palliation through the use of less-toxic regimens, and not a futile search for complete remissions through aggressive regimens such as CAP and CHAP. The immediate use of cisplatin is not better than a course of therapy that begins with a less toxic agent.

Platinol

In three tests comparing various platinum-containing regimens, response rates were typically between 40 and 80 percent. For example, the best responses were obtained in a group of 26 patients at Indiana University who received cisplatin + doxorubicin + cyclophosphamide. Eleven of the patients achieved a complete response, and another eleven had a partial response. Median survival for the entire group was just over two years—27.5 months—which happens to be the best results achieved in any such trial.

It is commonly said that women with stages II, III or even some stage IV cancers "have an excellent prognosis" (356). What is odd is that although this can be inferred indirectly, it cannot readily be seen through *direct* evidence.

Valid comparisons do not exist

To provide direct evidence would require a strict comparison of drugs versus untreated controls. "Randomized comparisons with untreated controls of immediate vs. postponed therapy are lacking," Abel points out, "and today they would probably no longer be accepted since ethical committees consider the use of chemotherapy as unrenounceable," i.e. obligatory. No one can now ethically administer (and no patients would probably participate in) a chemo-vs.-placebo trial.

Dose-effect studies

You will remember that one of the three kinds of direct evidence is the dose-effect study. This shows whether survival increases when more of the drug in question is given. But for ovarian cancer there have been no pure, randomized dose-effect studies. One study purports to analyze such data (229). It was seriously flawed, since it was based on a collection of quite incomparable studies (3).

Another small study compared survival of patients receiving high-dose cisplatin vs. low-dose cisplatin + chlorambucil. The high-dose patients had 24 months survival vs. 14 months for the low-dose patients. This advantage was confined, however, to a certain subgroup of stage III patients. And the treatment had to be interrupted for 15 out of the 46 high-dose patients because of "intolerable toxic effects," but for only 3 in the low-dose arm.

In a larger Dutch trial five-year survival rates were 32 percent for patients receiving high-dose therapy vs. 18 percent for those receiving low doses. The seven-year survival rates were 25 percent vs. 12 percent. But, again, there was much greater toxicity in the high-dose group, a point to which we shall return.

As with other studies in ovarian cancer, there is a strong impression of benefit from the chemotherapy, but a disturbing lack of proof.

Non-randomized studies

Belief in the effectiveness of chemotherapy in ovarian cancer must therefore be based primarily on non-randomized comparisons. Yet we know that such comparisons are of questionable value in an assessment of any therapy (3).

For example, claims are sometimes based on historical controls. In the U.S., five-year relative survival was 36.5 percent in the period 1974 to 1976, and had increased to 41.8 percent by 1983 to 1990, a statistically significant difference (323). And age-adjusted mortality in the U.S. had dropped from 8.4 deaths per 100,000 women in 1973 to 7.9 in 1991. However, what is strange is that *all* of that improvement took place by 1980. This would seem to militate against the idea that this improvement was due to intensive chemotherapy.

Cured by chemo?

And contrary to many published and widely accepted statements by oncologists, there no proof that patients with advanced ovarian cancer can actually be cured through chemotherapy. Supporters of chemotherapy point to the fact that 60 percent of women who have a complete remission (CR) are alive five years later. But what happens at this arbitrary five-year mark? As far as the tumor is concerned, nothing special. Survival curves do not flatten after five years (3). Instead, the estimated death rate from tumor-related causes beyond the five-year point is about ten percent per year (76,283,284). In addition, survivors in the most advanced cases, so-called FIGO stage IV, are still very rare.

Publication bias

It is particularly important to recall the prior discussion of publication bias. When one looks at the *published* clinical trials, combination chemotherapy for ovarian cancer looks better than single-agent chemotherapy. However, when investigators added in the unpublished trials, this significance completely disappeared (343).

Significant toxicity

Any life extension in ovarian cancer must be weighed against the very significant toxicity associated with the use of platinum-containing drugs and paclitaxel (Taxol). Cisplatin can typically cause kidney damage, hearing loss, severe nausea, vomiting, and nerve damage (363). Carboplatin appears less toxic, but may also cause significant bone marrow toxicity. For many patients, either regimen can be a grueling experience.

Comedian Gilda Radner, who received chemotherapy for her eventually fatal ovarian cancer, recalled her horror at its initial effects:

"A few mornings later, I woke up and the first thing my eyes focused on was hairs all over my pillowcase....Looking down onto the bathtub floor while I was shampooing, I saw it was covered with hair swirling toward the drain—my hair. I was devastated" (312).

Radner's best-selling book, *It's Always Something*, did much to bring the effects of chemotherapy to public attention. Kathy Hitchcock who rejected chemotherapy for her own cancer, remarked, "I felt that in the name of modern medicine, Gilda Radner was put into a torture chamber more diabolical than anything dreamt up during the Inquisition" (26).

Taxol

In addition, a great many hopes have been invested in paclitaxel (Taxol), which has been approved by the FDA for the treatment of ovarian cancer. In a 1989 Johns Hopkins study, doctors did in fact see an objective response (tumor shrinkage) in 30 percent of ovarian cancer patients who had failed to respond to conventional treatments. Patients were treated every 22 days with varying doses of Taxol given as a 24-hour infusion. They were also given premedication to avoid the acute hypersensitivity reactions that are sometimes seen with this drug. Forty such patients were evaluable for response. Twelve of these patients "responded to Taxol for periods lasting from 3 to 15 months." It remains to be seen how durable such responses will be, however.

Quality of life in ovarian cancer

Virtually none of the studies on the effectiveness of chemotherapy in ovarian cancer incorporates any measure of quality of life. Defenders of chemotherapy point out that ovarian cancer patients often have troublesome symptoms, such as ascites (accumulation of fluid in the abdominal region) as well as painful masses. Therefore, the use of combination chemotherapy, which tends to relieve these symptoms, could result in an improvement in life quality (102).

This may very well happen, but it remains unproven by rigorous studies. One must also weigh against this putative advantage a decrease in quality of life by the toxicity of the drugs, particularly cisplatin and paclitaxel (Taxol).

Other kinds of cancer

This completes our discussion of the four major kinds of adult carcinoma in which chemotherapy has at least been tested for effectiveness. As we have seen, the benefits in some cases appear real, but are quite limited in terms of actual survival advantage. Toxicity can also be considerable, even life-threatening.

But what about the other kinds of cancer? Does chemotherapy have any proven value at all in these? We shall discuss the situation in several dozen different kinds of malignancy below. In some of the relatively rare kinds of cancer of children and young adults, mentioned already, chemotherapy definitely provides a survival advantage—even a cure. But for the vast majority of cancers, the situation is much more problematical.

Adrenal gland

The adrenal gland is located adjacent to the kidneys and is involved in the fight-flight reaction to stress. Oddly, there are only about 150 to 300 cases of primary adrenal cancer each year in the United States. In stage III adrenal cancer, the tumor has already migrated outside the gland into the fat but has not yet involved the regional lymph nodes or adjacent organs. In stage IV, the tumor has metastasized. A drug called mitotane (o,p-DDD or Lysodren), a close relative of the insecticide DDT, is used as an "adrenal cytotoxic agent" and by poisoning the gland reduces the amount of hormone produced by the tumor. It may also retard tumor growth.

According to one small study, 7 out of 8 patients receiving high amounts of the drug had objective responses and significantly longer rates of survival (377). This treatment "may lead to partial or complete remissions lasting several months," according to Malin Dollinger, M.D. (104). But "the difference between efficacy and toxicity is small," he wrote, and the side effects of the drug can be drastic (285).

Seventy-nine percent of those who take mitotane tablets suffer from gastrointestinal toxicity (anorexia, vomiting, diarrhea), 50 percent have neuromuscular toxicity, and 15 percent experience skin rashes. Although there have been claims of a few long-term survivors (195), most patients relapse and the five-year survival rate is less than one percent (285).

Anus

This type is also rare and constitutes only one to two percent of all large bowel cancers. In recent decades, radiation and chemotherapy have helped reduce the extent of radical surgery needed in the treatment of this kind of cancer. In stage IV, however, in which the cancer has spread to the tail bone (sacrum), distant lymph nodes, or other organs, "there is no standard treatment" (328) and relieving symptoms becomes the only realistic goal. Towards this end, a combination of various drugs, usually including fluorouracil, is often given as a palliative and "may be a good salvage program." Nevertheless, there is no evidence that such treatments extend life and five-year survival is called "unusual" (327).

Bile duct

Bile duct (biliary) cancer causes 4,000 U.S. deaths per year. The staging system for bile duct cancer is different than for most cancers. Although a TNM staging system does exists, the main question to consider is whether the disease has spread beyond the bile ducts themselves to some vital organ of the digestive tract. It usually has, and by that point it is considered inoperable and untreatable by conventional means.

Some drugs, such as carmustine and doxorubicin, have caused partial responses in a limited number of patients. But "studies have not shown that chemotherapy can prolong survival," says Alan P. Venook, M.D., a San Francisco oncologist (380).

Nevertheless, mitomycin or fluorouracil (5-FU) are often given to patients. These may cause tumors to shrink and to help, in unspecified ways, about 25 percent of patients. Dr. Venook frankly admits that "even with tumor shrinkage, however, patients may not be better off after chemotherapy. The treatment has side effects and the tumor ultimately regrows" (380).

Bladder

In 1995, there will be an estimated 50,500 U.S. cases of cancer of the urinary bladder, with 11,200 deaths. Worldwide, this is the tenth most common malignancy. Ninety percent of bladder cancer in Western countries is of the "transitional cell type." About 30 percent of patients are discovered with distant metastases and about half the patients already have invasive tumors, from which distant metastases will eventually develop. With distant metastases, the five-year survival rate is less than two percent.

Much ado about nothing?

A number of drugs have been used against bladder cancer: cisplatin, methotrexate, vinblastine, doxorubicin, cyclophosphamide, and 5-FU. Combinations are said to achieve response rates of 30 to 50 percent, sometimes as high as 80 percent (369). Various drugs or combinations of chemotherapy are often employed. Thirty-five to 70 percent of patients are said to "respond" with tumor shrinkages. Alan Yagoda, M.D. further claims that 15 to 35 percent have "a complete tumor regression that sometimes lasts more than five years" (399).

However, a 1994 British review looked at the use of chemotherapy for metastatic transitional cell carcinoma. Over time, it has been shown that there has been no meaningful impact on survival in such cases (326). In the words of one chemotherapist, it may be a case of "Much Ado About Nothing" (313).

"No demonstrable impact has been discerned," the British reviewers noted, "from single agent-, or most combination-chemotherapy regimes on the poor survival of patients with metastatic disease" (326). For superficial bladder cancer the situation appears to be much the same: "Neither [chemotherapy's] exact role nor the optimal dose or schedule of administration have been established. To date, no dramatic differences in efficacy between the agents commonly used for intravesical chemotherapy...have been appreciated" (370).

Toxicity

Chemotherapy for bladder cancer can be extremely toxic. Cisplatin and methotrexate can be damaging to the kidneys and doxorubicin to the heart. "Even when kidney and heart functions are normal," Dr. Yagoda warns, these programs "can result in major complications in almost a quarter of the cases" (399).

In order to give ever-increasing doses of these and other drugs, doctors are now using agents such as filgrastim (Neupogen), which stimulates blood cell production. The resultant decrease in bone marrow toxicity enables them to give higher doses of chemotherapy.

Adjuvant use

Chemotherapy is also sometimes used as an adjuvant to facilitate more conservative surgery. One group of doctors has reported that they could use less extensive surgery (in an operation called a "partial cystectomy") when they also gave high-dose methotrexate, and achieve the same survival figures (351). Another approach is to use chemotherapy, especially cisplatin, first and then to use surgery to consolidate any good response. Long-term survival rates from this approach are not yet available, however.

In the 1980s, there were excited reports of high response rates, raising expectations of great benefit. But randomized trials of chemotherapy given in addition to surgery have failed to show any advantage to this approach (320,341).

In general, readers should be highly skeptical about "results" in bladder cancer that are achieved in small, uncontrolled trials at single centers, no matter how prestigious the hospital or the doctor. About such uncontrolled trials, the British reviewers commented on the likely "role of chance in determining treatment outcome in small series of patients..." with bladder cancer (326).

Brain and central nervous system

There will be an estimated 17,200 U.S. cases of brain and central nervous system (CNS) malignancies in 1995, with 13,300 deaths (11). Males are somewhat more likely to be afflicted than females. There are two main types of primary malignant brain cancer, *anaplastic astrocytomas* and *glioblastoma multiforme*. These are life-threatening, but rarely metastasize (59). Other forms of brain cancer—*medulloblastoma, germ cell tumors, malignant ependymoma,* and *choroid plexus carcinoma*—

do commonly spread via the central nervous system.

The five-year survival rates for brain and other nervous system cancers range from 42 percent when the disease is localized to one percent when there are distant metastases (323).

Surgery and radiation are considered the standard treatments, although the complete removal of the tumor is difficult to attain, since it would often result in significantly impaired mental and nervous system function. Corticosteroids are used to decrease swelling.

There are vast complexities to the treatment of this disease.

Overall, "the role of chemotherapy in the treatment of childhood brain tumors is increasing," according to NCI scientists (303). However, the basic story was summed up in a few words by a prominent San Francisco neurosurgeon:

"The chemotherapy of brain tumors has consistently been among the most disappointing failures in clinical oncology, achieving at best only short-term palliation" (160).

According to the European (EORTC) reviewers, "chemotherapy [of malignant glioma] adds little if anything to postsurgical irradiation in terms of median and/or mean survival" (176).

Astrocytomas

These tumors are usually treated with surgery and radiation. In Grade III, however "the cure rate is low." Five-year survival is in the range of 10 to 20 percent, although there is no indication that treatment actually prolongs survival or cures anyone.

The chemotherapy of astrocytoma is entirely experimental and is limited by the fact that many cytotoxic drugs are stopped by the blood-brain barrier. Carmustine is sometimes used, as well as cisplatin, vincristine, procarbazine, hydroxyurea, cytarabine, cyclophosphamide, flourouracil (5-FU), and etoposide.

Glioblastoma multiforme

"Glio" is a very rapidly growing form of brain cancer. Five-year overall survival is less than five percent. It is said that "chemotherapy and improved surgical technique" have been responsible for "doubling the survival time (once the tumor is diagnosed) and improving the quality of life" (104). The chapter in Dr. DeVita's textbook that deals with brain tumors states categorically that such treatment "increases both TTP (time to progression) and survival" and lists a dozen trials of irradiation and chemotherapy for patients with anaplastic astrocytoma and glioblastoma multiforme. But these are comparisons of different chemotherapy combinations and do not provide information comparing drugs to good supportive care.

In any case, survival with treatment appears to be approximately a year for 50 percent of those with relatively high performance scores (so-called Karnofsky scores of 60 or better) (230).

Some other forms of brain tumor are treated with surgery and/or radiation, apparently with some success, but chemotherapy is not usually involved in this. These include brain stem gliomas, medulloblastomas, meningiomas, and primary central nervous system lymphoma.

"For recurrent glioblastomas and anaplastic astrocytomas," one surgeon has written, only about 20 percent have remissions lasting a year. But "adjuvant chemotherapy is even less effective, adding little time, if any, to the survival of patients who undergo surgery and radiation for these tumors" (160). In fact, he considers even the experimental use of chemotherapy in such cases ill conceived:

"[D]espite the localized nature of almost all malignant brain tumors, the principal experimental thrust in their treatment has been the application of systemic chemotherapy—a modality for which the traditional target has been disease that spreads beyond its site of origin. The emphasis on systemic chemotherapy for malignant brain tumors seems particularly misguided...."(160).

Medulloblastoma

The five-year disease-free survival rate for low-risk patients is 77 percent and for high-risk patients, 39 percent. For this type of brain cancer, it has been said, "the usefulness of chemotherapeutic agents is regrettably restricted," since the bone marrow is usually so damaged by previous radiation to the head and spine that patients cannot "tolerate the challenge of systemic chemotherapy" (160).

There have been at least 15 small trials using single chemotherapeutic agents against this kind of brain cancer, and another 10 using combinations. Some of these claim high rates of responses (e.g., 7 out of 7 with cyclophosphamide). Yet, amazingly, none of these studies offered information on the *durability* of the responses. Nor is there any logical reason to use combination chemotherapy, since there have still been no well-founded studies that compare single vs. multiple drug use (230).

Cervix uteri (see also uterus)

The cervix is the "neck" of the uterus (womb). In 1995, there will be an estimated 15,800 new U.S. cases of cancer of the uterine cervix, and 4,800 deaths. Worldwide, the death rate ranges from a high of 15.9 in Mexico to a low of 0.9 in Italy. Distant metastases are infrequent. In general, treatment is based on radiotherapy. In advanced cases, methotrexate + doxorubicin or bleomycin + mitomycin are said to bring about response rates of over 40 percent. But once again, there are no indications from randomized studies that survival is improved by doing this (364).

Supporters of chemotherapy point to increasing survival rates for this kind of cancer. The U.S. mortality rate was 5.2 deaths per 100,000 in 1973 but just 2.9 per 100,000 in 1991 (323). But such historical improvement should probably be attributed to the early detection of the disease with the Pap smear test as well as improved hygiene, rather than to chemotherapy.

There are two studies purporting to show a benefit from adding chemotherapy (the drug hydroxyurea) to radiotherapy in the treatment of large tumors that do not have distant metastases. In one randomized study of 97 patients, the median survival of patients receiving chemotherapy was 19.5 months compared to 10.7 months in the group receiving radiation therapy alone. But the survival of patients at two years was almost the same (187).

Another small study purported to show a major increase in five-year survival using a combination of radiation with chemotherapy over the use of radiation alone (94 percent five-year survival for the combination group vs. 53 percent in the radiation-alone group) (301). Not only was this study small, but it lost credibility when the authors were found to have excluded several deaths that occurred in the chemotherapy group, which they classified as unrelated to the tumors (3).

Choriocarcinoma

Choriocarcinoma is one of what are called the gestational trophoblastic diseases. These are a spectrum of growths that include the benign hydatidiform mole and the locally invasive mole. "Chorio" is the most malignant outgrowth of pregnancy, and involves the transformation or overgrowth of vital cells called trophoblasts. In a sense, then, it is not really a cancer of the adult patient, but of her fetus. In full-blown choriocarcinoma, abnormal fetal cells spread throughout the mother's body, and if left untreated, can overwhelm her immune system, invade her vital organs (especially her liver and brain), and rapidly kill her.

By using methotrexate, dactinomycin, and other drugs given intramuscularly, chemotherapists have scored one of their indisputable triumphs. The drugs kill the fetus's essentially foreign cancer cells, thus saving the woman's life. It is an impressive victory. Sustained complete remissions are achieved in about 80 percent of patients (97).

It should not detract from this victory to point out that in a technical sense choriocarcinoma is not really curable at all, but remains 100 percent fatal *to the organism in which it developed*, namely the fetus. It is the malignant extension to the mother that is now routinely cured.

According to Cairns, this victory also has to be put in statistical perspective: the celebrated cure of this disease actually saves a total of 20 to 30 lives in the U.S. each year (60). The disease is said to be far more common in Latin America and in Asia (97).

For other reasons, choriocarcinoma is a poor model for the treatment of other cancers. Unlike choriocarcinoma, ordinary tumors do not originate in the cells of another creature. It is an order of magnitude more difficult to design drugs that can cleanly distinguish between the normal cells of the body and one's own home-grown malignant cells.

Esophagus

The esophagus is the tube that carries food to the stomach. In 1995, there will be an estimated 12,100 new U.S. cases of esophageal cancer, with 10,900 deaths (11). All forms of treatment have been of modest help here and chemotherapy alone or in combination is of little benefit. A combination of two drugs (fluorouracil + cisplatin) is sometimes used before surgery to shrink the tumor. Fluorouracil + mitomycin have also been tried. In Stage III, fluorouracil + interferon is said to have shown significant activity, but five-year survival is less than ten percent.

In Stage IV (with distant metastases), there is no standard treatment; however, chemotherapy is sometimes used for its alleged palliative effects. Five-year survival is called "unusual."

Gall bladder

Cancer of the gall bladder is a relatively rare and aggressive disease. It is generally without symptoms until it reaches an advanced stage. In early stages, treatment basically consists of surgical removal of the organ (cholecystectomy). Part of the liver and the lymph nodes may also be excised. Advanced disease is sometimes treated with radical surgery as well, but such use is considered controversial. As to chemotherapy, no studies have shown that chemotherapy can prolong survival. In advanced gall bladder cancer, in fact, no standard therapy has been established. Two-year survival remains under one percent.

Head and neck

Squamous cell carcinoma of the head and neck is a diverse category encompassing several different kinds of cancer. Chemotherapy has been used for three main purposes: as a neoadjuvant, to shrink tumors before surgery; as adjuvant therapy; and as a palliative.

In general, high-dose chemotherapy for head and neck cancer has failed to show any survival benefit over low-dose chemotherapy (382). Nor has combination chemotherapy shown any advantage over single agent therapy.

One study using 24-hour continuous infusions purported to show a slight survival benefit (161). But this study was marked by a number of irregularities. After randomization, 10 out of 38 patients were excluded from the study as inappropriate. By excluding some or all of their failures from the list of "evaluable patients" these doctors may have made their results appear better than they really were.

Further bias was caused by the fact that the control category was eliminated from the test after doctors performed an interim analysis of the results. However, survival in another therapy group, using the drugs cisplatin + bleomycin, was actually worse than it had been in the above control group, but this second study was not ended.

Oropharynx

Five-year survival is 14 percent for cancers of the tonsils and 20 percent for the back of the tongue. While the primary treatments are surgery and radiation, neoadjuvant chemotherapy is often used to shrink tumors, facilitating these other treatments.

Nasopharynx

Five-year survival is 15 to 25 percent. Treatment is complex, mainly surgery and radiotherapy, not chemotherapy.

Larynx

Treatment is mainly surgery and radiotherapy. Chemotherapy may be given for palliation. Dr. Alvan Feinstein and colleagues at Yale University have published some statistics on this kind of cancer. They found that survival correlates not just with the standard TNM classification, but even more so with the patient's symptoms. *How the patient is functioning can be used as a major prognostic factor even within what appears to be the same stage of the disease.* In 193 patients, he wrote, the total five-year survival was 66 percent, ranging from 78 percent for stage I to 35 percent in stage IV. But when patients were analyzed by the severity of their functional impairment, the corresponding rates ranged from 83 percent in the most functional group to just 15 percent in the least functional, regardless of their TNM stage (300).

Hodgkin's disease (see lymphoma)

Kaposi's sarcoma

Kaposi's sarcoma (KS) was once a rare tumor of older men. Now it has become relatively common, because of its association with AIDS (so-called epidemic KS). It is not considered curable, but long-term survival can occur both with and without treatment. Single agents such as doxorubicin, bleomycin, and vinblastine have been tried. Although some disease-free survival has been seen with this ABV regimen compared to doxorubicin alone, no difference in overall survival was seen (138). Also, according to the NCI, no benefits have been seen for interferon with chemotherapy regimens as compared to single agents.

Although new drugs and combinations are always being tried, treating epidemic KS with drugs involves several major problems.

"One concern about using very aggressive therapy is that the treatment might further depress the immune system," according to Dr. Dollinger. Although the classic form of KS is said to be "highly responsive" to vinblastine, there is no information on how AIDS-related KS is likely to respond. Vincristine is also in use and side effects are said to be "remarkably low" (104).

In the early days of AIDS, says Dollinger, combination chemotherapy regimens were nearly always used. "They fell into disfavor because of the high death rate from drug toxicity...." With the less toxic drugs, treatment is often continued indefinitely.

The "AIDS drug" zidovudine (AZT) has no effect on the extent or progression of Kaposi's sarcoma (104).

For *AIDS-related lymphomas*, similar problems apply: treatment is difficult because of the problems of HIV infection. For this AIDS-related condition there is also no clear consensus on any standard form of chemotherapy.

Kidney and ureter

In 1995, there will be an estimated 28,800 new U.S. cases of kidney cancer in the U.S., with 11,700 deaths. The standard drugs used in its treatment are vinblastine and the nitrosoureas, carmustine and lomustine. These are said to produce tumor regressions in five to ten percent of cases. In stage IV, five-year survival is five percent. At this point, says Dr. Yagoda, "participation in an experimental protocol...would be very appropriate" (399).

Sixty patients with metastatic kidney cancer were given the experimental cytotoxic drug lonidamine with high-dose tamoxifen for over six months. Results at the Hannover University Medical School in Germany suggest that lonidamine and high-dose tamoxifen do not cure this disease but are "moderately effective" in widespread kidney cancer if the "treatment intention is palliative" (353).

Leukemia

This large group of cancers of the blood generally affect the white blood cells (leukocytes). One type of leukemia, acute lymphocytic leukemia of children, is *successfully treated with chemotherapy*. This needs to be acknowledged and recognized, so that people who read this book, and might understandably be disillusioned with chemotherapy, will not pass up an effective treatment, when it is appropriate.

However, there are many misperceptions about leukemia and its cure. Although primarily thought of as a childhood disease, leukemia actually strikes *ten times as many adults* as children. Results in adults are not nearly as good as in children.

In 1995, an estimated 25,700 Americans will develop leukemia, and 20,400 will die of it. Thus, despite public perception that leukemia is readily curable through chemotherapy, the fact is that about four out of five patients still die of their disease. The highest rates in the world are in Hungary, New Zealand, Denmark, the former Czechoslovakia, Israel, and Italy (10).

There are many types of leukemia, with a corresponding array of names. These can be categorized into two great groups, the acute and chronic, which occur in almost even numbers each year.

In earlier decades, leukemia was often classified as a "blood dyscrasia" or one of cancer's "allied diseases," rather than a true malignancy.

Acute leukemia is characterized under the microscope by the proliferation of the "blast forms" of blood cells that refuse to become mature. These proliferate and crowd out the more mature cells of the bone marrow or blood.

Chronic leukemia involves cells that do in fact mature, with only a few blast forms present. Although they appear normal they do not function as such. Diagnosis is made on the basis of symptoms (an inability of wounds to heal, etc.) rather than by microscopic analysis. As the name "chronic" implies, these blood diseases are naturally slow-moving, and even untreated patients can survive for years with this condition.

The treatment of leukemia depends on the type, although chemotherapy is involved in almost every kind.

In preleukemia (the so-called myelodysplastic syndrome), the goal of treatment is to control the disease, not eradicate it. The drug of choice is hydroxyurea, an orally administered antimetabolite, which can cause low blood counts, nausea, vomiting, diarrhea, iron loss, loss of appetite, and constipation. The purine analog thioguanine and the alkylating agent busulfan may also be used.

Some investigational attempts are being made to "push" such premalignant cells towards normality. However, if this condition develops into full-blown leukemia, then standard chemotherapy is initiated.

Acute leukemias

Acute leukemia itself is subdivided into an array of different types. About 80 percent of adult leukemia patients have one of these types: acute myelogenous, acute myeloblastic, acute monocytic, acute monoblastic, acute myelomonocytic, or premyelocytic leukemia.

Acute lymphocytic leukemia (ALL)

Acute lymphocytic leukemia (sometimes called acute lymphoblastic leukemia, and both abbreviated as ALL) is sometimes also called "childhood leukemia" because it usually affects a younger population. Treatment is generally effective for ALL and the prognosis is good. Patients with this type of cancer have a higher response to chemotherapy than do those with other kinds of leukemia.

Many drugs are used in its treatment, including vincristine, doxorubicin, cyclophosphamide, cytarabine, and the hormone prednisone. This disease is also one of the few uses for a one-time wonder drug, L-asparaginase.

There is no need for us to go into great depth on treatment for this disease. However, we will note that the toxicities of this "cure" can be horrendous. As just one example, a 1990 article in *Pediatrics* noted the high frequency of what it called "acute mental status changes" in children undergoing therapy.

"Children with acute lymphocytic leukemia," it noted, "were more prone to having seizures (61 percent), while children with non-acute lymphocytic leukemia were almost equally likely to have encephalopathies [brain diseases, especially associated with alterations of brain structure, ed.], strokes, or seizures" (103).

We will thus repeat our position that these treatments, while effective, can be barbaric in their side effects, and the need for nontoxic substitutes is almost as urgent as it is in the case of adult cancers.

Acute myeloid leukemia (AML)

In AML, standard treatment usually involves daunorubicin and cytarabine. Cytarabine is another of those drugs noted for its very high ability to cause nausea and vomiting. Additional drugs, such as ondansetron (Zofran), are given in an attempt to control such side effects. In addition, chemotherapeutic drugs kill normal and leukemic cells almost equally and so patients may require blood transfusions.

Experimentally, doctors are using the anti-tumor antibiotic, mito-xantrone, as well as etoposide, amsacrine and/or carboplatin in the treatment of this cancer.

Chronic leukemias

There are also several different kinds of chronic leukemias, which vary in their aggressiveness and thus in their treatment. Ironically, chronic leukemias, while slow-growing, tend to be more deadly than many treatable acute leukemias.

Chronic lymphocytic leukemia (CLL)

Patients are not automatically treated. Although less aggressive than acute leukemia, often progressing slowly, these cases are not curable by conventional means. When it is treated, chlorambucil and cyclo-phosphamide are generally used, either singly or in combination with prednisone. Experimentally, fludarabine is also being used.

Chronic myelogenous leukemia (CML)

This affects the myeloid cell line rather than the lymphocytes. Hydroxyurea and busulfan are most commonly used. Patients are often placed on allopurinol (Zyloprim), which prevents the high levels of uric acid often associated with this condition. Bone marrow trans-plantation is often considered as a possibility in this disease.

Hairy cell leukemia

Hairy cell leukemia is more like a chronic than an acute leukemia. Since 1985, it has been treated with interferon-alpha, allegedly with a 70 to 80 percent success rate. Treatment is administered for two years. When it is discontinued, however, about a quarter to a third of patients develop the disease again.

Lymphomas

Like leukemia, lymphoma is also divided into two basic types:

Hodgkin's disease

Hodgkin's disease (HD) is a cancer of the lymphoid system, which will afflict 7,800 Americans in 1995, with 1,450 deaths. It is named after its discoverer, Thomas Hodgkin (1798-1866), who described its features in 1832. HD is another condition that is *frequently cured by either radia-tion or chemotherapy.* MOPP (mechlorethamine + vincristine + procar-bazine + prednisone) is the protocol of choice, but half a dozen other protocols are also in use.

Although Dr. DeVita states that "Hodgkin's description was the first of a distinct malignancy of the lymphatic system" (96), in the older literature HD was usually not considered a true cancer.

Hodgkin's disease is radically different than most other kinds of cancers. For example, the "tumors" of Hodgkin's disease often contain very few Reed-Sternberg cells, the standard marker for this type of cancer. Also, the scarring of lymph tissue seen primarily in this type of tumor is a very uncharacteristic response to cancer.

Hodgkin's disease is also unusual in that it spreads in an orderly progression from one lymph node area to another, usually from the neck to the collarbone, from there to the arms, and then to the chest. This is quite different from the unpredictable distant spread of most cancers and also makes it atypical.

Its features were so unlike those of other malignancies that in the past most doctors were convinced that it was a kind of deadly infection, possibly caused by corynebacteria. Others thought it was related to tuberculosis. Another name for HD was "pseudo-leukemia." Today it is believed there is a strong association with the Epstein-Barr virus and "considerable epidemiologic evidence in support of an infectious cause, particularly a virus, has been found" (96).

HD frequently attacks adolescents and young adults, but about 75 percent of newly diagnosed patients can be cured with radiotherapy and/or combination chemotherapy. Radiation is the treatment of choice in Stage I or Stage II patients with good prognoses.

Chemotherapy is employed in all other stages. Treatment generally consists of MOPP, ABVD, or a modified combination of the two, which involves the use of seven separate toxic agents. Patients are said to have prolonged disease-free survival on combination chemotherapy. Patients whose cancers recur after such chemotherapy, however, are not generally cured, but long remissions have been reported.

Five-year survival ranges from about 90 percent in favorable Stage I, to 60 to 80 percent in Stage IIIB or Stage IV cancers.

The treatment itself carries an increased risk of leukemia, in about one to five percent of patients receiving MOPP, usually within four years of the initiation of treatment. Other cancers may also result from the radiation treatment. For example, French scientists report seeing six cases of cancer of the breast following treatment for Hodgkin's disease (88).

The conquest of Hodgkin's disease is certainly another triumph of modern medicine. But because of its peculiarity and relative rarity, it is unwarranted to extrapolate from the successes with HD to other cancers. And yet, oddly, that is exactly what has happened. The high-dose, multi-drug approach used in HD is routinely taken as the model for treating the more common solid tumors of adults. This is spelled out by two Stanford University oncologists:

"The systematic approach to the pathologic diagnosis, staging, treatment strategies, and clinical trials that have been developed for Hodgkin's disease over the past 30 years serves as a model for all modern cancer therapy" (167).

But, as Dr. Jerry Z. Finkelstein, M.D. (writing in the same book) has said, "Childhood cancers are different from those of adults. The growth pattern is different and the tumors react differently to treatment" (121). Over 80 percent of cancers in adults are carcinomas (epitheliomas), whereas over 90 percent of the tumors seen in children are malignancies of bone, blood vessels, muscles, or supporting tissues.

Non-Hodgkin's lymphoma

All other cancers of the lymphoid system are grouped together as non-Hodgkin's lymphomas. This is a far larger category, accounting for 50,900 new U.S. cases in 1995, with 22,700 deaths. These are classified according to their growth rate: low-, intermediate-, and high-grade tumors. They are also divided into B and T cell type cancers.

Low-grade tumors are very slow growing, yet incurable by conventional means. The long-term outcome has not been seriously affected by chemotherapy. The treatments for advanced disease are controversial. They go from no initial treatment to combination therapy with one or more of the following regimens: CVP, C-MOPP, or CHOP.

Intermediate- and high-grade tumors are treated aggressively with chemotherapy and radiation. This is said to "cure" 70 to 80 percent of patients with limited disease and to "eradicate" the cancer in about 50 percent of those with advanced disease. Patients with favorable prognoses are said to enjoy a cure rate that approaches 80 percent.

Again, standard treatment may include CHOP in the favorable stages I and II. For all other cases, in addition to CHOP, either M-BACOD or the very intensive ProMACE-CYTABOM is employed. Five-year survival is said to be about 40 to 50 percent, although for people over 60 the statistics are not as good. In the high-grade tumors, patients with extensive disease have generally not done well with conventional therapy, with a reported 20 percent five-year survival. Bone marrow transplantation is increasingly common, but no definitive results are available.

Liver

In 1995, there will be an estimated 18,500 new U.S. cases and 14,200 deaths from liver cancer (including biliary passages). Around the world, liver cancer is one of the most common malignancies. Not much needs to be said: in general, it has not been successfully treated with conventional cytotoxic drugs.

"Chemotherapy," says San Francisco oncologist, Alan P. Venook, M.D., "may result in tumor shrinkage, but this does not necessarily prolong survival" (381). Doxorubicin may shrink the tumor somewhat, but the side effects of this drug can be so devastating that it "may leave patients in a worse condition even if the tumor shrinks." Infusion devices that feed toxic drugs directly into the liver will bring about a higher rate of regression (up to 50 percent) in some patients. But "the therapy is difficult to give and extremely toxic to an already damaged liver" (381).

One new treatment technique is called "chemo-embolization." This involves the administration of a combination of chemotherapy and colloidal particles directly into the liver via its main hepatic artery. Although tumors will shrink in about 50 percent of cases it needs to be emphasized that "prolonged survival has not been proven" (381).

In advanced disease, Dr. Venook again emphasizes "no standard treatment is known to prolong survival." Chemotherapy is said to possibly relieve the pain of large liver masses (although this must be weighed against the side effects of the drugs). Two-year survival is less than 5 percent.

Malignant melanoma (see also skin)

While most skin cancers are not life-threatening, there is one form that is very serious indeed. That is malignant melanoma (literally, black tumor). There will be an estimated 34,100 new cases in 1995, with 7,200 deaths. Melanoma can spread to each and every organ of the body. It can spread from mother to fetus. It is also one of the most common tumors to metastasize to the spinal cord and brain.

In its early stages, it is said to be highly curable through surgery. A wide excision is believed to be best, with a clearance of 3 to 5 cm from the borders of the tumor. Once it has penetrated deeply into the skin or has reached the blood or lymphatic systems "it is often impossible to cure," according to University of Southern California professor Malcolm S. Mitchell, M.D. (104).

Chemotherapy is widely used for melanoma, however there is little if any evidence that it extends life. It is said that it can cause "responses" in 40 to 64 percent of cases. Initially, the most commonly used agents were the drug dacarbazine and the immune agent, BCG. However, in the first three trials on patients with regional disease "no definite effect was shown" (227). Even proponents admit that the percentage of complete response is low and the duration of response short.

In stage II, with lymph node involvement, various studies have been done after lymph node dissection (surgery). Between 1978 and mid-1984, 13 trials were published on chemotherapy and/or immunotherapy for this type of cancer. Some of these failed to have a control arm, whereas others failed to randomize the patients. "Taking into account randomized patients," says Dr. Ferdy Lejeune in the European (EORTC) review, "there was no positive adjuvant effect with any of the treatments" (227).

In fact, assessing all 51 trials that were done between 1979 and 1984, Dr. LeJeune concluded that "none of the attempts to improve the results in melanoma have been successful. Combination chemotherapy was in general not better than dacarbazine alone, and immunotherapy, when used as an adjuvant to surgery or chemotherapy, was a complete failure" (227). LeJeune adds "it was surprising to find so many trials without appropriate control arms, especially in adjuvant studies, and so many reports that were published too early to evaluate."

High response rates?

Since the mid-1980s, other studies have been done, but remain experimental at best. A 1991 study from Canada claims that in stage II, the addition of levamisole increased remission durations and survival times (311). High-dose chemotherapy as part of bone marrow transplantation has been said to cause high "response rates." The cost of this treatment is very high and involves from four to six weeks in the hospital. After all that, the average remission is just four months and 15 to 25 percent of the patients, by Dr. Mitchell's estimate, die of the treatment itself (104).

For stage II patients, NCI concludes that "autologous bone marrow transplantation with high-dose chemotherapy has not been shown to improve survival (259).

In stage III melanoma of the extremities, experimental protocols center around not just the use of adjuvant vaccines and immunostimulants, but what is called hyperthermic (heated) perfusion of chemotherapy (136,137). These are not yet proven to extend life, however.

In stage IV, results have generally been disappointing. According to NCI, "the objective response rate to dacarbazine or semustine is approximately 20 percent" (277). These responses generally last less than six months, and once again combination chemotherapy has no proven advantage over single drugs. When given at doses requiring bone marrow transplant support, alkylating agents such as melphalan or thiotepa produce an objective response rate of approximately 50 percent, but with responses generally lasting less than 6 months.

In a study at the M.D. Anderson Cancer Center in Houston, previously untreated patients with metastatic melanoma received the experimental drug paclitaxel (Taxol) by an IV drip. All patients first got various agents to prevent allergic reactions. Three of the 25 patients had a partial response (PR). In addition, four patients had some objective regression of the tumor size.

These "failed to qualify" as partial responses, but the scientists called some of these responses "durable." In addition, partial responses lasting more than three months were seen in 4 of 12 melanoma patients treated with Taxol in a study at Albert Einstein Cancer Center (PDQ, 2/18/95).

A discussion of immunotherapy lies beyond the scope of this book. Although advanced melanoma is relatively resistant to treatment, several biologic response modifiers and cytotoxic agents have been reported to produce objective response rates of around 20 percent.

Dr. Steven Rosenberg of NCI has described three complete and three partial responses among 34 evaluable patients following treatment with LAK cells and high-dose bolus IL-2, and all three complete responders were disease free between 11 and 32 months of follow-up. The treatment can be highly toxic, however.

"Although continuous infusion high-dose IL-2 + LAK may be less toxic than bolus high-dose IL-2 + LAK, the continuous infusion schedule appears to be less effective," says NCI (277).

Malignant mesothelioma

This is a malignant tumor of the chest lining and abdominal cavities. About 2,000 new cases are diagnosed in the U.S. every year. Generally, people who develop this kind of tumor have a history of having been exposed to asbestos.

Even orthodox authorities admit that malignant mesothelioma is not generally curable, although a few surgical cures have been reported in a number of patients with very localized tumors.

Treatment is generally directed at symptomatic relief. Chemotherapy has been extensively tested in the treatment of this disease, mostly to no avail. Doxorubicin, cyclophosphamide, and cisplatin are said to be "active." So, too, are 5-azacytidine (a cytidine analog), fluorouracil (5-FU) and high-dose methotrexate with leucovorin rescue factor. In addition, combination chemotherapy may yield higher response rates, especially when containing doxorubicin.

For localized malignant mesothelioma, five-year survival has not been determined since cases are rare. For peritoneal mesothelioma, survival beyond one year is equally unusual.

Multiple myeloma

This is a cancer of the blood, specifically of the plasma cell, a B lymphocyte responsible for producing antibodies. There will be 12,500 new cases in 1995 with 10,300 deaths. Two-thirds of the people with multiple myeloma experience bone pain. Chemotherapy is used extensively in this disease. The major controversy is whether to give a single alkylating agent such as melphalan together with prednisone, or to give a combination of alkylating agents. The "objective response" rate with melphalan + prednisone is about 50 to 60 percent. The various combinations can produce an "objective response" rate of 75 percent. Nevertheless, even orthodox sources admit that the survival is about the same: two to three years.

"Almost all patients with multiple myeloma who do respond to chemotherapy will eventually relapse if they do not die of some other disease in the meantime," says Robert A. Kyle, M.D., of the Mayo Clinic.

If chemotherapy is stopped, the patient generally relapses quickly. If chemotherapy is continued longer, the patient may suffer bone marrow damage and develop acute leukemia. The immunotherapeutic agent alpha interferon is increasingly being used in the treatment of this disease.

For recurrent or refractory myeloma the PDQ system states: "Chemotherapy should be given to all patients with advanced or symptomatic disease" (277). There is no indication, much less proof, that this results in increased survival.

Oral (mouth)

There will be an estimated 28,150 new cases of cancer of the mouth (oral cavity) in the U.S. in 1995 (11). About 8,370 Americans are expected to die of it in 1995. The U.S. incidence is twice as high in men as in women.

Worldwide, the death rate varies from a high of 14.7 per 100,000 among Hungarian men to 0.6 among women in Greece. Other countries with high rates include Hong Kong, France (males), Singapore, and Luxembourg (10).

Tobacco and excessive use of alcohol are considered the main risk factors for this kind of cancer. Vitamin A deficiency is also considered a risk factor for oral cancer, while a high dietary intake of beta carotene and antioxidants, as found in fruits and vegetables, is considered protective (133,134,231).

Surgery and/or radiation are the mainstays of treatment, but they are beyond the purview of this book. There have been reports of the use of chemotherapy as an "induction therapy" to reduce the amount of tissue that needs to be removed during surgery (397). But because of its ineffectiveness, chemotherapy is basically not used in the treatment of this disease.

Pancreas

There will be 24,000 new U.S. cases of pancreatic cancer in 1995 and 27,000 deaths! One of the reasons for the high death rate is that symptoms generally do not occur until this particular kind of tumor has already spread. This is the fifth leading cause of cancer death in the United States. Overall survival figures are still extremely poor (only three percent are alive at five years) regardless of the treatment used.

It is particularly disturbing that the number of cases of pancreatic cancer is increasing steadily, particularly in the industrialized countries. Exposure to petrochemical compounds and solvents are believed to be one factor contributing to this increase.

In stage I adenocarcinomas, when the cancer is confined to the pancreas or has spread to just the adjacent tissues, the three-year survival rate is 15 percent. This may be misleading, however, since according to Abel, the five-year survival rate for all stages combined is only one to two percent (3). Median survival time for all patients is approximately six months from initial diagnosis.

Despite these generally dismal survival figures, an increasing number of patients are receiving chemotherapy alone or in combination:

Treatment of Pancreatic Cancer in U.S. Hospitals

Year	Surg. & Chemo	Surg. Rad. & Chemo	Chemo
1985/86	9.9	4.7	12.1
1991	13.4	3.3	12.9

Thus, nearly 30 percent of all patients received some form of in-hospital chemotherapy for this cancer. The standard treatment for early stage pancreatic cancer remains surgery and the disease is said to be sometimes curable by these means. About 90 percent of pancreatic tumors can no longer be removed surgically; when they are, the operation is considered extremely difficult and dangerous and 5 to 30 percent die on the operating table. In stage IV, when the cancer has already spread to distant sites, such as the liver or lungs, the three-year survival rate is only two percent.

Ninety percent of all pancreatic cancers are *adenocarcinomas* and most of these occur in the same portion of the gland that produces the pancreatic enzymes. Other, rarer kinds of pancreatic cancer are *islet cell carcinoma, adenosquamous, undifferentiated, small cell carcinomas, cystadenocarcinomas*, and *lymphomas*.

Chemotherapy studies

It is sometimes claimed that chemotherapy is in fact becoming effective in the treatment of pancreatic cancer (169). Three controlled studies have been done to assess the value of single-agent chemotherapy in prolonging life in pancreatic cancer. None of them was positive. In the first, a median survival of 44 weeks was seen vs. 9 weeks in the controls. But this study was flawed. In 14 out of the 40 patients in this study there was lack of proof (histological confirmation) that the cancer had in fact spread (246).

A second, larger study of 152 male patients was completely negative (129). In fact, the group receiving the chemotherapy (5-FU + CCNU) lived a shorter time, a median survival of three months (median) compared to 3.9 months for the controls. A smaller study in 1986 also failed to show any survival value to chemotherapy (338).

Combination therapy?

Cytotoxic drugs given in combination are said to result in response rates of over 30 percent. This would seem to be a strong argument for combination treatment, and it is on the basis of such studies that many pancreatic patients are aggressively treated. Yet, once again, there is little evidence that such therapy correlates with an increased life span.

All indirect evidence, like the direct evidence, is entirely negative. There is no marked or consistent difference between the various chemotherapeutic regimens. Survival rates continue to be extremely poor, regardless of what drugs chemotherapists direct against this tumor.

Islet cell carcinomas

These are relatively rare tumors of the pancreas, for which the primary treatment remains surgery. Some chemotherapeutic drugs are said to be "active" against these tumors, although we know of no controlled trials proving that they increase survival time of patients. Some of these drugs include doxorubicin, cyclophosphamide, dacarbazine, fluorouracil, streptozocin, and etoposide.

Gastrinomas

The primary treatment is surgery plus other (non-chemotherapeutic) drugs, such as the anti-ulcer medication, Tagamet. Occasionally, drugs for islet cell carcinoma are suggested as well. Five-year survival is 65 percent.

Insulinomas

These are mostly benign growths. Fluorouracil + streptozocin or somatostatin/octreotide (Sandostatin) are sometimes given. Five-year survival is 60 percent.

Parathyroid

The parathyroid glands are located in the neck, two on each side of the thyroid. Unless they malfunction, one is unlikely to ever know they exist. While benign tumors of the parathyroid gland are fairly common (an incidence rate of between 1 and 5 per 1000 persons), malignant carcinomas are unusual, only afflicting about one percent of these cases. And even so, cancers of the parathyroid are relatively benign. However, since the parathyroid glands produce a hormone that has the important job of regulating calcium levels in the blood, this tumor can lead to a condition called hypercalcemia, which is difficult to control and may eventually be fatal.

Surgery is the treatment of choice for both localized and metastatic disease. For patients with advanced disease, dacarbazine, as well as 5-FU + cyclophosphamide have been used. Five-year survival in such patients is about 20 percent.

Penis

Cancer of the penis is rare, each year afflicting about one or two men out of 100,000 in the United States. It is almost never seen in those who are circumcised as babies. Most penis cancers are non-fatal squamous cell carcinomas of the skin. Some, however, are melanomas. Occasionally, the deep tissues develop sarcomas.

While the five-year survival rate is almost 100 percent in stage I, by stage IV, when it has spread to distant sites, it is less than 5 percent. There are a number of experimental chemotherapy protocols in use.

Regimens for urethral or penile carcinomas are similar to those used in bladder cancer. Because of the limited number of cases, there is little documentation of responses. For squamous cell tumors of the penis, some activity of cytotoxic drugs has been demonstrated in about half of the relatively few patients treated with single agents (bleomycin, methotrexate, or cisplatin).

Combinations include cyclophosphamide + bleomycin + cisplatin. At M.D. Anderson Cancer Center in Houston they have used mitomycin + cisplatin. There were ten responses out of 12 patients, but the duration of these responses was only 5.9 months (98).

Pituitary

This is another relatively rare form of cancer. Ninety percent of the time tumors of this gland at the base of the brain prove to be benign. Sometimes, however, by putting pressure on the nerves to the eye even benign growths can cause a decrease in vision or blindness. Hormonal deficiencies can also develop. Standard treatment includes surgery and radiation, not chemotherapy. Radiation is said to control the growth of these tumors in more than 90 percent of the time. However, the drug mitotane, a close relative of the insecticide DDT, is sometimes used. The drug bromocriptine has also been used to reduce symptoms by lowering the levels of prolactin in the patients. A new drug, CV205-502, is said to be helpful in patients who no longer respond to bromocriptine. There is no evidence of significant life prolongation with any of these agents.

Prostate

Cancer of the prostate is the most common cancer among American men, overtaking both lung and colorectal cancer in the 1980s. This disease mainly affects men over 65. About 244,000 American men will be diagnosed with prostate cancer in 1995, and 40,400 will die from it (11). Prostate cancer is not to be confused with another common problem affecting this gland, benign prostatic hyperplasia (BPH), which may cause overlapping symptoms.

The death rate from prostate cancer varies from a high of 22.5 per 100,000 in Switzerland to a low of 3.8 in Japan and 2.6 in Hong Kong. Other countries with high rates include Norway, Sweden, Uruguay, and New Zealand (10).

The disease of half of the patients is limited upon discovery to the gland itself; in the other half it has already metastasized.

More accurate diagnostic techniques (such as the prostate-specific antigen, PSA) are leading to earlier detection and therefore more cases. However, the value of such screening is controversial. "[T]he benefits to the public" of such screening "is uncertain," says Dr. Norman R. Zinner. "Most men with prostate cancer will die from other illnesses never knowing they had the problem" (406). In fact, according to one report, over 30 percent of men above the age of 50 have latent prostate cancer—8 million American men in all.

Prostate cancer is the second most commonly diagnosed cancer in men. It is one in which surgery, radiation and hormone drugs (not cytotoxic agents) are the treatments of choice.

Treatment of Prostate Cancer in U.S. Hospitals

Year	Prostatectomy	Hormone Drugs
1985/86	13.9	20.6
1991	26.7	18.8

Since there were about 200,000 new U.S. cases in 1994, this would amount to 37,600 cases treated in the hospital with hormonal drugs. There was a surprising, albeit slight, decline in the use of hormones in the years in question. (There is no category given for combinations of drugs and surgery and/or radiation.)

Meanwhile, this did not mean a trend towards less aggressive treatment. Quite the opposite. Radical prostatectomy—the complete surgical removal of the prostate gland—almost doubled (from 13.9 to 26.7 percent), a trend that many observers have found alarming. Is this medically warranted? Prostatectomy rates vary widely, especially by geographical region. For instance, a man in New England has a 14.9 percent chance of receiving this operation, while the same patient in the Pacific region has a 26.4 percent chance—almost double. Yet their cancers are the same; it is the doctor's proclivities that are different.

In localized tumors, surgery and/or radiation are generally used. In what is called Stage D, the cancer has spread to the lymph nodes and distant sites and "is rarely curable." Nevertheless, the tumor might be relatively slow growing. The five-year survival is said to be 55 percent in stage D-0; 40 percent for D-1, and 35 percent for D-2 and D-3.

In advanced prostate cancer, such as Stage D, hormone therapy is used to slow the growth of the tumor and reduce symptoms. Some of these hormones are DES, an antiestrogen flutamide (Eulexin), other hormone-like agents (like leuprolide), and progesterone-like agents, such as Megace. A so-called chemotherapeutic-hormonal agent, estramustine phosphate, is also being used experimentally when patients no longer respond to the usual hormone-modulating drugs.

Certain chemotherapy regimens are being tried experimentally. For example, the drug suramin has been tested against carcinoma of the prostate (273). The "response rate" in two Phase II trials ranged between 33 and 40 percent. But in the first study the incidence of severe side effects was over 80 percent. In the second, it was said to be 20 percent (273). "Its final role in the treatment of carcinoma of the prostate remains to be defined," according to three doctors prominent in the field (163).

At least a fourth of all males over the age of 70 who die of other causes have small cancers of the prostate upon autopsy. The number may be even higher: according to one classic study, 40 percent of those aged 70 to 79 had prostate cancer, and 67 percent of those aged 80 to 89 (11).

Steady improvement?

The five-year survival rates for all stages combined have "steadily improved," according to the ACS, and "in the past 30 years have increased from 50 percent to 80 percent" (11). U.S. government statistics confirm that the five-year relative survival rate was 43 percent in the period 1950 to 1954 and 81.3 percent in 1983 to 1990 (10).

Yet oddly there has been *no* major advance in the treatment of prostate cancer since the introduction of hormone therapy in the 1940s. How is this possible?

What is happening is this: the national incidence of prostate cancer rose rapidly from 878 per million in the early eighties to an extraordinary 1,630 per million in 1991 (10). Even the ACS attributes this dramatic increase to "improved detection." In other words, with the emergence of the Prostate Specific Antigen (PSA) and other diagnostic tests, doctors could find little tumors that were lurking deep in the folds of aging prostates—find them, treat them and "cure" them.

"Further increased incidence is expected with widespread use of serum screening tests," says the ACS (11). However, by most accounts, fewer than ten percent of those tumors are destined to ever produce symptoms. Thus, medical science is now "curing" tens of thousands of prostate cases that would never have come to anyone's attention, if not for a well-coordinated campaign to find and eradicate them.

As Cairns states, "even if the campaign saved no lives, the inclusion of these additional, non-fatal 'cancer' cases would inevitably increase the proportion of 'patients' who survive" (60).

The increased survival of prostate cancer patients is therefore not a triumph of cancer medicine of the same type as the successful treatment of many cases of childhood leukemia. On the contrary, it is mainly a statistical artifact, and ultimately the result of a kind of iatrogenic (doctor-caused) illness (191).

The inclusion of such cases, however, greatly inflates the "cure" figures. Lots more people are made into cancer patients, subjected to intensive treatment, and then thank their lucky stars that the doctors "found it in time" and "got it all." In reality, the great majority would never have known they had a problem if it hadn't been for the march of technology and the eagerness of doctors to extend the boundaries of their therapeutic domain.

Feeble voices are sometimes raised to rein in this artifactual "epidemic" of prostate cancer. But Cairns goes further: he suggests that "similar artifacts probably affect the survival rates for many other types of cancer, particularly cancer of the breast." For that reason, it has become a principle, at least among many cancer epidemiologists, "that the comparison of the survival of patients in different eras is not in general an acceptable measure of therapeutic success..." (60).

In prostate cancer, a great many claims are based on such dubious distinctions.

Rectum (see colorectal)

Sarcomas of the bone and soft tissue (see also Kaposi's sarcoma)
Sarcomas are a class of relatively rare and unusual tumors that start either in the bone, cartilage, fat, connective tissue, or muscle. There are nearly two dozen different kinds of sarcomas. Altogether, about 7,000 cases of soft tissue and 3,000 cases of bone sarcoma are diagnosed each year in the U.S. They account for about one percent of all adult tumors, but 15 percent of childrens' tumors.

Age is a determining factor in who gets what kind of sarcoma. *Soft tissue sarcoma* tends to afflict adults between 40 and 60 years of age. *Chondrosarcoma* primarily affects those in their 50s. *Osteosarcoma* mainly affects teenagers. *Ewing's sarcoma* is found mainly in children aged five to nine and then again in young adults aged 20 to 30. *Rhabdomyosarcoma* affects youngsters aged one to three.

In addition to surgery and radiation, chemotherapy is used very extensively in the treatment of some sarcomas. For the children in particular, this approach has been quite successful. However, it is generally agreed that the kind of doses required to achieve a good chance for "cure" often produce very serious side effects.

Single agents used include doxorubicin, cyclophosphamide, high-dose methotrexate (with leucovorin rescue), ifosfamide, dacarbazine, vincristine, dactinomycin, etoposide, as well as some investigational drugs. There are half a dozen commonly used combinations, such as

CyVADIC.

In adult soft tissue sarcomas, chemotherapy can be used as a primary treatment; along with radiation; as an adjuvant; or as a palliative. Such usage generally involves combinations that include doxorubicin and dacarbazine, as well as other agents. Ifosfamide is sometimes added to the regimen.

Standard therapy is not curative for adults, however, and so patients are often asked to join experimental clinical trials.

Skin (see melanoma)

Overall, the most common kind of cancer is that of the skin. Over 800,000 cases of basal cell and squamous cell skin cancers are diagnosed in the U.S. each year, with 2,100 nonmelanoma skin cancer deaths (11). Since such skin cancers do not generally metastasize, they are not included in the U.S. statistics of cancer incidence. (If they were, U.S. cancer incidence would top two million per year!)

Skin cancer is increasingly rapidly in our society. It once was seen mainly in older people, but is increasingly found in people in their twenties and thirties. The most common forms are basal cell cancers (BCC) and squamous cell cancers (SCC).

There are currently nine different treatments used for this disease, most often including surgery or radiation. However, sometimes the drug fluorouracil (5-FU) is applied directly to the lesion. This blocks DNA synthesis, cell growth, and eventually kills the malignant cell. It can therefore be used to treat superficial basal cell cancers. When applied twice a day for four weeks or more, 5-FU causes an inflammatory reaction, which heals after treatment. 5-FU has also been used internally, with unknown effectiveness, in the treatment of those occasional skin cancers that have spread to distant sites.

In addition, there are at least three drug-like treatments that are under development:

Retinoids, which are similar to vitamin A, are also being tried experimentally in the treatment of skin cancer. They are said to demonstrate an "adequate cure rate" when used to treat basal cell cancers. In squamous cell cancers, there was a 70 percent response rate in one study.

If the retinoids are not synthetic analogs, but are given in their natural, vitamin form, there are minimal side effects.

Alpha interferon, a biological response modifier, has been injected directly into basal cell cancers, with apparently good results, as well. It also has good cosmetic results. There are side effects, however, including short-term fever, chills, muscle aches, and headaches.

Photodynamic therapy combines a directed light with a type of drug called a photosensitizer. The most common photosensitizer in use today is called HPD. This is injected intravenously and then the tumor is exposed to different colors of light, usually red or blue-green. This initiates a reaction that kills the tumor.

Small intestines

Although the small intestines comprise the longest portion of the gastrointestinal tract, malignant cancers are much less common there than they are in the esophagus, the large bowel (colon), or the rectum. In fact, only 1.5 percent of all GI cancers are found in the small intestines.

Small intestinal tumors can be adenocarcinomas, sarcomas, carcinoid tumors, or lymphomas. Altogether, there will be approximately 4,600 cases in the U.S. in 1995, with about 1,120 deaths (11). People over 60 have an elevated incidence of this disease. There are a number of intriguing theories about why cancer is less common here, but no firm answers.

Cancers of the small intestines are generally slow to grow or to metastasize and are usually treated by a simple surgical removal of the tumor. Chemotherapy is used for tumors that for one reason or another cannot be removed surgically or have already metastasized. The chemotherapy employed is generally 5-FU + leucovorin; 5-FU + streptozocin; or 5-FU + carmustine. Five-year survival is 20 percent for adenocarcinoma. Biological response modifiers, such as alpha interferon, are also in the process of being evaluated.

Combination chemotherapy is the standard treatment for some advanced cases of *lymphoma of the small intestines.* If the disease is localized, or when 12 or more of the nearby lymph nodes are removed and show no signs of disease, there is a 40 percent chance of five-year survival. In diffuse lymphoma the five-year survival rate is 25 percent.

Solid tumors of childhood

Under this heading are found a number of rare conditions that while actually distinct, are generally grouped together. Altogether, the incidence of these solid tumors of childhood adds up to about 3,500 cases per year. They not only primarily afflict infants and children, but grow very quickly and are thus more susceptible to drugs that kill dividing cells. And indeed, in this category chemotherapy has scored some impressive successes.

Many of these illnesses are associated with congenital syndromes, anomalies, malformations, or recessive genetic defects. For that reason, it is unwarranted to extrapolate from these successes to more common cancers.

In addition, in some locales, childhood cancers appear in clusters, and may be the result of viruses, chemical pollution, or possibly electromagnetic exposure. There have been notable outbreaks of such childhood cancer in Niles, Illinois and Woburn, Massachusetts. In the latter case, the cancer cluster was eventually tied to chemical pollution of the water supply (97).

Wilms' tumor

This is a rare form of kidney cancer that affects children. It becomes even less common after the age of seven. Annual incidence is seven cases per million children under the age of 16. In 1991, there were 460 new cases in the U.S.

Wilms' tumor is usually first discovered as a mass in the abdomen. Conventional treatment involves surgery, radiation, and chemotherapy. In the 1960s, it was found that the drug dactinomycin diminished the growth of this tumor. Now vincristine, doxorubicin, cyclophosphamide, and cisplatin are also used. Response rates are as high as 63 percent. In stage IV, three of these four drugs may be used.

The "cure" rate—in this case, measured as a four-year (not the standard five-year) relapse-free survival—ranges from around 90 percent in stage I to 55 percent in stage IV. As might be expected, toxicity is often drastic. In one study, there were at least 17 toxic deaths from leukopenia (destruction of white blood cells) and liver failure. At one time, ten percent of infants were dying from the side effects of the drugs, but dosages are now said to have been cut back by 50 percent, with a concomitant decrease in toxicity.

Neuroblastoma

This disease is said to "represent frustration and hope to those who treat cancer in children." Despite many complete responses, cure is still elusive and recurrences are common. Chemotherapists believe, however, that because of these responses "there is an implicit promise of more effective and less toxic treatments" (303).

The annual incidence is 10 per million children, or about 525 new cases in the U.S. each year. For reasons unknown, it is especially found among African-American children. Neuroblastomas are similar if not identical to certain anatomical structures that are normal when seen in fetuses or very young infants.

Another peculiarity of neuroblastoma is that sometimes the disease will spontaneously regress. It can occur anywhere in the sympathetic nervous system, as well as the adrenal gland, the chest, or pelvis.

Treatment consists of surgery, radiation, and chemotherapy. The response rate is said to be 59 percent with cyclophosphamide, and combinations involving high-dose cisplatin, vincristine, and other drugs are employed. For high-risk patients, the survival rate is said to be 15 percent "despite several therapeutic approaches," (303) including bone marrow transplantation (BMT). But while BMT may increase survival, relapses continue to occur.

Retinoblastoma

In children, this is the most common primary tumor of the eye. There are 11 cases per million children under the age of five, or 200 new U.S. cases per year. Treatment is surgery or radiation; the role of chemotherapy is considered undefined. Some of the drugs used are vincristine, cyclophosphamide, doxorubicin and methotrexate. These produce short-term, mixed, or partial responses.

Stomach

In 1995, 22,800 Americans will be diagnosed with stomach cancer (gastric carcinoma), and 14,700 will die (11). Although it is considered highly treatable in its early stages, most cases are not discovered until they have already spread to nearby or distant organs.

Until 1945, stomach cancer was the leading cause of cancer deaths in the U.S. But, for reasons unknown, the incidence of stomach cancer has been decreasing in the United States, falling about 60 percent between 1930 and 1970. Oddly enough, the U.S. now has the *lowest rate* of stomach cancer in the world for both men and women (5.2 and 2.3 per 100,000). The rates in Costa Rica are over 10 times as high. Other countries with high rates are the former Soviet Union, Chile, Canada, and Japan.

What treatments are people actually receiving? The National Cancer Data Base (NCDB) figures contrast usage in the period 1985 and 1986 with that in 1991 (the latest date for which figures are available). The NCDB shows that the use of chemotherapy is increasing for this type of cancer, while the use of surgery (gastrectomy) was declining slightly.

Treatment of Stomach Cancer in U.S. Hospitals

Year	Surgery	Combinations	Chemo
1985/86	40.4	16.4	09.9
1991	37.8	17.8	11.8

Combination treatment in this case means either surgery with radiation; surgery with chemotherapy; or surgery with both radiation and chemotherapy. The use of this term in reference to stomach cancer introduces another element of uncertainty into the figures. For our purposes, however, let us hypothesize that two-thirds of those in this "combination" category received chemotherapy in addition to some other treatment. Of the 22,800 new cases, over 5,000 therefore are likely to receive some form of chemotherapy as part of their in-hospital treatment.

Clinical trials

There have been several randomized studies that directly addressed the problem of whether chemotherapy increased the survival of patients with advanced stomach cancer. Essentially the results of these studies are negative.

In 1969, Dr. Charles Moertel of the Mayo Clinic compared the effects of a combination of supervoltage radiation with chemotherapy (5-FU) vs. the effects of radiotherapy alone. There was a statistically significant difference in favor of the combination, but the difference was less than three months. Dr. Moertel himself conceded that 5-FU may only have compensated for a reduction in survival *caused* by radiation therapy (264).

In a 1979 study, scientists found that there was no difference between giving no treatment; radiation + 5-FU; or intravenous chemotherapy with thiotepa.

All chemotherapy regimens appear about equally ineffective. The "response rate" with single drugs is always around 20 percent. Up to 50 percent responses can be seen with combination chemotherapy (such as the FAM regimen). Such responses are usually just partial, however. In terms of length of survival, there is no evidence that combination chemotherapy is any better than single drug therapy.

Neither is there indirect evidence that survival of patients with gastric cancer is increased by chemotherapy. In short, there is no proof that chemotherapy prolongs survival in advanced stomach cancer. A 1986 review of the entire field concluded, "There is still therefore no therapy for advanced gastric cancer that can be recommended as standard treatment" (346).

According to Drs. Rosenbaum and Dollinger, "chemotherapy can offer significant palliation to some patients and long-term remissions are sometimes possible" (327). However, according to a 1987 prospective, randomized trial, there was no advantage in survival of adjuvant chemotherapy compared to patients who underwent surgery alone

(152). The five-year survival rate for stage IV stomach cancer remains less than five percent.

Testis

Cancer of the testis (also called germ cell cancer) accounts for about one percent of malignancies among all American males. There are about 7,100 cases per year, with 370 deaths—itself testimony to *the effectiveness of conventional therapy in this kind of cancer.* The five-year survival rate has gone from 63 to 91 percent in the last 30 years, mostly as a result of improved diagnosis and chemotherapy.

The treatment of testicular cancer represents an indisputable triumph of cancer medicine, albeit with a high price paid in toxicity and other side effects.

Testicular cancers are divided into two broad types: *seminomas* and *non-seminomas*. Seminomas make up about 25 to 40 percent of all testicular cancers. Such patients tend to be in their thirties. Non-seminomas affect even younger men.

Most non-seminomas are composed of various unusual cell types. In some cases they resemble choriocarcinomas (the malignant tumors of pregnancy). Some testicular cancers are mixtures of germ cell tumors, embryonal cell carcinomas, yolk-sac tumors, teratomas, and other tissues. Obviously, we are dealing here with atypical growths, even for cancer.

Surgery (orchiectomy) is employed in almost all cases, followed by radiation and/or chemotherapy. In stages II and III there is an array of possible combinations. These can include mixtures of drugs such as cisplatin, vinblastine, etoposide, and bleomycin.

In early stages, standard treatment with surgery and/or radiation is effective. Five-year survival is said to be between 95 and 100 percent. Since most cases will not relapse after this initial therapy, some doctors advocate a wait-and-see attitude towards further treatment.

Even in stage III, survival is said to be 90 percent. Such patients are given cisplatin and etoposide (EP), or the same two drugs with bleomycin added (BEP). Doctors continue with the treatment until they have totally obliterated all signs of cancer—"only complete response is acceptable," according to Dr. Alan Yagoda (399).

Some chemotherapists seriously argue that their successful treatment of testicular cancer "can serve as a paradigm for the multimodal treatment of solid tumors" (112). But it is unreasonable to extrapolate from chemotherapy's successes in treating these rare, atypical tumors to the general run of advanced carcinomas.

Thymus

Cancer of the thymus, a gland in the middle of the chest, is a rare condition. The types of cancers here can include lymphomas, germ cell tumors, carcinoids, carcinomas, and thymolipomas. Malignant thymoma is the most common tumor of this organ. In stage I, the tumor is generally non-invasive and is treated by simple surgical removal. If there is no evidence of spread, there is no further therapy.

Sometimes adjuvant radiotherapy or chemotherapy is suggested to prevent spread. The recurrence rate for this type of cancer is two percent. Even in advanced stage II and III, surgery and/or radiotherapy are the standard treatments. Five-year survival is said to be 54 percent.

Chemotherapy is experimental, with cisplatin + doxorubicin + vincristine + cyclophosphamide said to produce a 91 percent "response rate" in one study. In another, a combination of cisplatin + doxorubicin produced a 70 percent response rate (104).

Thyroid

Cancers of the thyroid gland comprise about one percent of all malignancies in the U.S. There will be about 13,900 new U.S. cases in 1995, three quarters of them in women. Invasive thyroid cancer is uncommon. But about four percent of the population develop thyroid nodules, most of which are benign, but have to be biopsied nonetheless.

There are three basic kinds of thyroid cancer. Papillary thyroid cancer is generally treated by surgery. In advanced stages, radioactive iodine is frequently used as treatment. Stage IV is treated with chemotherapy, but five-year survival is said to be less than 20 percent.

Follicular thyroid cancer

Treatment generally consists of surgery and/or radiation, including radioactive iodine, called I-131. In stage IV, chemotherapy is sometimes used experimentally, but five-year survival is said to be unusual.

Medullary thyroid carcinoma

Surgery is the treatment of choice and there generally is no benefit to chemotherapy.

Anaplastic thyroid carcinoma

This is an extremely aggressive tumor. Radiation therapy combined with doxorubicin (which acts as a radiation sensitizer) is the standard treatment. Given weekly, doxorubicin is said to shrink some of these tumors. Patients usually die within one year of diagnosis, however, the average being six months. Five-year survival is around five percent.

Primary lymphoma of the thyroid

Treatment is approximately the same as for other non-Hodgkin's lymphomas, i.e., they are treated with aggressive "third-generation" combination chemotherapy.

Uterus (see also cervix uteri)

In 1995, there will be an estimated 32,800 new U.S. cases of cancer of the corpus (body) of the uterus, usually of the endometrium (lining). The endometrial types represent about 95 percent or more of incidence. In addition there is also a rare kind of cancer of this organ —uterine sarcoma.

The death rate from (non-cervical) uterine cancer ranges from a low of 1.4 per 100,000 in Hong Kong to a high of 13.7 in Ecuador (10). Other countries with high rates include Venezuela, Mauritius, and Cuba. Those with the lowest rates include Australia, Iceland, and Singapore (10).

Endometrial Carcinomas

This cancer of the lining of the uterus is the most common gynecological malignancy. It accounts for about one percent of all malignancies in women. There will be 15,800 invasive cases and 65,000 carcinomas in situ (i.e. non-invasive) cases in 1995.

In the early stages, the five-year survival rate is high (83 percent in 1985). However, this tumor is sometimes first diagnosed in a late stage, and over 4,800 women die from it each year.

Treatment generally includes surgery and/or radiation. Chemotherapy is being evaluated for treatment of late-stage disease. These studies are looking at the role of such drugs as doxorubicin, mitoxantrone, cisplatin, cyclophosphamide, carboplatin, and various hormones as adjuvant treatments for stages Ib and beyond.

In stage III, five-year survival is said to be up to 30 percent. But in stage IV, it drops to around five percent.

Link with tamoxifen

Tamoxifen (Nolvadex) is now being used as a second-line treatment for cancer of the endometrium. But, ironically, in 1991 scientists at the Karolinska Hospital in Stockholm, Sweden reported "an increased incidence of endometrial cancer associated with long-term adjuvant tamoxifen." This follows reports that tamoxifen stimulates the female genital tract and has a "mainly estrogenic effect" on these tissues.

"An increased incidence of endometrial cancer may limit the usefulness of tamoxifen for benign indications," the Swedish scientists reported in the *Annals of the New York Academy of Sciences.* In their opinion, the improvement in both recurrence-free survival and overall survival in early breast cancer "probably outweighs" the increased frequency of uterine tumors (126).

However, they warn that the possibility of stimulating the growth of hidden groups of cancer cells "should be considered when tamoxifen is used in the treatment of endometrial cancer" (126).

To investigate the link between tamoxifen and endometrial cancer, doctors at Maimonides Medical Center in Brooklyn, New York screened their breast cancer patients who had received tamoxifen for at least 12 months. Seventy such patients were interviewed and endometrial biopsies were obtained from 38. Seven (18 percent) had hyperplastic (i.e. pre-cancerous) changes, ranging from simple through complex abnormal changes with atypical cells.

Uterine sarcomas

These are far rarer and account for only 1 to 5 percent of all uterine malignancies. Surgery and/or radiation is the standard treatment. Cytotoxic drugs are often recommended as well, "although there is no definite proof of increased survival with adjuvant chemotherapy...," according to Dr. Jeffrey L. Stern, M.D., a gynecological oncologist (356). In advanced cases, five-year survival is said to range between 0 and ten percent.

Vagina and vulva

Carcinoma of the vagina is relatively rare: it strikes 2,000 American women per year, or one to two percent of all gynecological malignancies. Most of these are squamous cell carcinomas. Adenocarcinomas and melanomas also occur. Carcinoma in situ, a non-invasive stage, is said to be 100 "curable" through radical surgery, or with lasers, 5-FU cream, or implants of radioactive cesium.

In stage I through IVa tumors, chemotherapy may be given simultaneously with radiation. Investigation regimens include mitomycin + 5-FU with or without cisplatin. In stage IVb, in which the tumor has spread to distant organs, no treatment is curative and five-year survival is less than ten percent. A number of chemotherapy regimens are routinely tried. These include either cisplatin or carboplatin or the ICE regimen.

These same drugs, plus fluorouracil (5-FU), vincristine, etc. are being used in various investigational protocols.

Melanomas of the vagina are treated very aggressively, but the prognosis is poor. One regimen used is dacarbazine + cisplatin +

cyclophosphamide + tamoxifen.

Conventional treatment consists of radical excision of the vulva, with removal of lymph nodes as well. In some cases, radiation and/or chemotherapy are being used as a substitute for this drastic, but seemingly curative, treatment. Drugs used include 5-FU + mitomycin + cisplatin. In advanced cases, the prognosis is poor. Five-year survival is five percent when there are lung metastases, but up to 25 percent when metastases are limited to the pelvic lymph nodes. In stage IVb "there is no standard chemotherapeutic regimen" (356).

CHAPTER NINE

Quality of Life

‏

OFTEN, WHEN APOLOGISTS FOR chemotherapy are forced to admit that drugs rarely extend actual survival, they fall back on another argument: that at least they have a "palliative" effect on the patient.

"It was frequently emphasized in the correspondence," wrote Dr. Ulrich Abel about his communications with oncologists, "that the primary goal of chemotherapy is purely palliative..." (3).

So the question arises, Does chemotherapy really "palliate"advanced cancer? Does it improve the patient's quality of life?

The word "palliate" is derived from the Latin word for cloak. To palliate is to cover over or moderate the intensity of an illness, short of a cure (372). Yet the whole study of quality of life in cancer, quite frankly, is in a shambles.

A fuzzy notion

Most of us have a fuzzy, but common sense, notion of what makes up a better quality of life. In cancer it generally includes increased appetite; the ability to carry on normal activities; relief from depression and anxiety when these are present; relief from the symptoms of the disease itself; or from the toxic side effects of the therapy.

However, there is no cookie-cutter definition. For one thing, a sense of life quality is culturally determined: different cultures or even individual doctors use different criteria to measure this elusive concept. It "depends very much on the specific culture area," wrote one doctor. It may also differ greatly among countries, even such otherwise similar societies as the U.S., Great Britain and Germany (174). So, when scientists talk loosely about quality of life, they often are comparing different things.

"As yet," Abel wrote, "no consensus has been reached on the selection of relevant variables, the method and time of data collection, or the weighting and combination of the parameters" (3).

Quality of life also differs for different individuals. Some can endure severe pain but are unable to put up with the slightest nausea. Others can take all kinds of unpleasant side effects so long as their pain is alleviated.

Every attempt at a simple definition so far has come up short, probably because quality of life is a multidimensional thing, incorporating differences based on the patient's expectations and background.

It is striking that the person most concerned, the patient, is rarely consulted on whether the treatment really does improve his or her quality of life. Alvan Feinstein, the Yale epidemiologist who has done so much to clarify biases in research, forcefully made this point:

"Because quality of life is a uniquely personal perception, denoting the way that individual patients feel about their health status and/or nonmedical aspects of their lives, most measurements of quality of life in the medical literature seem to aim at the wrong target. Quality of life can be suitably measured only by determining the opinions of patients and by supplementing (or replacing) the instruments developed by 'experts.'" (139).

Or, as Dr. Feinstein and his colleagues wrote in another context, "Ask patients what they want." (398). Yet, ironically, that rarely happens. For example, for some chemotherapists, tumor shrinkages or a few months' extra survival are everything; the quality of that extra time is rarely considered. Yet a study has shown that in a hypothetical situation 20 percent of healthy volunteers would choose radiation instead of surgery for laryngeal cancer, even though they were told it might result in a shorter period of survival (257).

The reason they gave is that radiation affords the patient a continued ability to speak normally, whereas surgery robs the patient of his or her normal voice. In this instance, patients and their families—those on the "receiving end" (73)—routinely valued quality of life higher than did their doctors.

Oncologists often justify the use of cytotoxic drugs on the grounds that they decrease tumor-related complaints. The burden of proof rests with the advocates of chemotherapy when they say that these drugs can and do palliate cancer. Impressive anecdotes are offered to support this view. But anecdotes are not proof. "The clinician has the duty," said Abel, "to furnish proof that cytotoxic treatment improves quality of life; it is not the critic's task to demonstrate the absence of evidence" (3).

There are in fact several reasonable goals that palliative chemotherapy might accomplish. One is to shrink a tumor that is pressing on a nerve, in order to decrease pain and increase mobility. Another is to shrink a disfiguring tumor, say, of the head and neck region. Yet another is to decrease effusions building up in the lungs or elsewhere, or painful paraneoplastic syndromes (cancer-related symptoms not directly attributable to the local effect of the tumors).

As legitimate as these goals are, it is important to note that these complaints are seen in only a relatively small fraction of all the patients actually administered palliative chemotherapy.

Astonishingly, given the extent to which cytotoxic drugs are being used, there have been no randomized studies yielding clear evidence of an improvement in quality of life through chemotherapy.

Subjective well-being is rarely measured in most trials. In the case of non-small-cell lung cancer, for instance, Dr. Elaine M. Rankin remarked that although "treatment may not alter the survival of patients....it may result in considerable symptomatic benefit leading to an improvement in the quality of life." Yes, it may. But does it do so? In NSCLC there is no proof. "Unfortunately," Dr. Rankin continues, "there are few reliable objective measurements of the quality of life to enable documentation of such improvements. Further work to establish such criteria is urgently needed" (314).

If chemotherapy really improved the patient's quality of life, one suspects there would be myriad studies showing this. The reason there are practically none has to be the obvious one—chemotherapy is not a palliative for most patients and in fact *diminishes* their quality of life.

In a few cases in which chemotherapy seems to improve life quality, there is an ironic dimension to this achievement. Doctors strive to achieve a "remission" with highly toxic drugs. When they finally achieve this temporary remission they stop giving the drugs. Thus, the treatment finally comes to an end, thereby automatically improving the patient's quality of life.

False hope?

Another attempt to prove the value of chemotherapy hinges on the question of hope. Doctors say that the mere administration of such drugs instills an otherwise despondent patient with fresh hope. This is independent of any question of the drugs' effectiveness.

"Expressed bluntly," said Abel, "this remark amounts to saying that patients may experience an improvement of their psychic well-being by a toxic therapy only because the truth regarding their prognosis is withheld from them" (3). Over the decades, there has been a blistering critique of alternative practitioners for allegedly purveying exactly this kind of pseudo-treatment. It is branded "false hope." But, once again, oncologists grant themselves a license they are not willing to afford others.

Even if we were to agree that in selected cases patients do experience an improvement in quality of life after chemotherapy, this alone is still not a compelling argument in its favor. Why? Because such improvements must be weighed against *all* the side effects in the *entire* patient population being treated. Otherwise, said Abel in a memorable analogy, the argument has the same structure as a recommendation for gambling based on the profit of the winners.

A decrease in the suffering of a few does not justify increasing the suffering of the many.

The same point was made about the interleukin-2 trials at NCI. Medical ethicist Prof. George Annas pointed out that "more than 80 percent of the patients did not do any better and they actually did worse. They died harder. That's not irrelevant. We always tend to concentrate on the survivors, but we've got to make the point that more than 80 percent had terrific side effects and didn't get any measurable increase in longevity" (*New York Times*, 3/23/94). And, as Prof. Martin F. Shapiro commented, the "revelations about the apparent ineffectiveness of the experimental cancer drug interleukin-2 are but the tip of an iceberg of misrepresentation" (340) and misunderstanding about cancer drug treatments in general.

Side effects are the Achilles heel of the chemotherapy establishment. If noted at all, they are often understated. One technical reason for this is a "subtle and hardly avoidable" bias built into the way data is reported. Patients who suffer and who are doing worse tend to be increasingly under-represented in the statistics. This is because they die earlier. We know of no attempts to correct the results of clinical trials for this kind of bias (3).

Wait-and-see strategy

One limited area in which quality of life has sometimes been examined is in studies of the relative value of immediate vs. deferred chemotherapy in lung cancer. And a 1971 study showed no difference between patients receiving drugs immediately compared to those whose doctors took a wait-and-see attitude (107).

In a second study, the quality of life in patients in the wait-and-see group was actually better. And while the control of symptoms until death may have been better in the group receiving chemotherapy, this was at the cost of an accelerated death rate within the first two months of the study (221).

Finally, in a study of the CAMP regimen vs. the single agent lomustine, scientists simply found no difference in quality of life between the two groups. The authors of that report concluded, "Such treatment for patients with unresectable non-small-cell lung cancer with minimal symptoms should not be considered beneficial until well-controlled trials demonstrating improvement in the quality of life or a survival advantage" (220). Such studies have still not been done.

Another often-quoted study of breast cancer patients purports to show that those receiving continuous chemotherapy have a better quality of life than those getting intermittent therapy (no survival benefit being seen in the trial). This conclusion was based on patient questionnaires. The authors gave a boost to the notion that chemotherapy improves quality of life:

"Those concerned about the toxicity of chemotherapy will find reassurance that continuous treatment was perceived by our patients as providing a better quality of life during chemotherapy for metastatic breast cancer"(74).

However, patients who were receiving continuous chemotherapy made more visits to the hospital than patients receiving just intermittent drugs. Such intensity of patient care will often improve a patient's mental outlook. Some patients may also have answered the questionnaire in a way designed to please the physician—an involuntary influence by the doctor.

In addition, questions about quality of life were not put to the patients during the early phases of the trial, when symptoms tend to be worse, but rather at the conclusion of each three-week cycle.

This timing led patients to concentrate their attention on the time that treatment was least intense, or when they were not receiving any treatment at all. For both these reasons, the results of this study are considered of little value with respect to quality of life (3).

Quality of life is rarely studied in relation to cancer chemotherapy and when it is the results are rarely positive. Our strong impression is that chemotherapy does not increase but diminishes the quality of life of most cancer patients.

Countering side effects

Various drugs, such as filgrastim (Neupogen), are now being used to decrease the side effects of chemotherapy. The important point is that such agents are not usually given to increase the patient's comfort, but to allow doctors to give even greater doses of cytotoxic agents.

In addition, since the late 1980s, many oncologists have begun using ondansetron (Zofran), as well as similar agents, to control the immediate nausea and vomiting following chemotherapy. But ondansetron is no miracle cure. It has side effects of its own, including headaches and constipation that may require further medication. Recent medical articles reveal:

• Even with ondansetron, vomiting remains a problem for 30 to 40 percent of chemotherapy patients (367). Even the manufacturer's scientists admitted (201) there had been no decent clinical trials comparing ondansetron to cheaper competitive drugs (367,368).

• Many patients whose immediate nausea was suppressed by the drug suffered what is called "delayed emesis" (vomiting) 24 hours or more later. "Delayed emesis does not seem to be adequately controlled by these drugs, and they may also lose some efficacy during multiple-day chemotherapy or after several cycles of chemotherapy" (1). In fact, "ondansetron yielded results equivalent to the prior placebo results," i.e., was not better than a sugar pill for this condition (215).

• Steroids, not ondansetron, "can still be considered the standard treatment" for patients treated with moderately nauseating chemotherapy (368). And "oral ondansetron is not superior to traditional anti-emetics for the prevention of nausea and vomiting caused by chemotherapy or surgery" (81).

• "Experience in the treatment of children is still limited" (407) but a two-year-old girl developed acute low blood pressure, slowing of the heart rate (bradycardia), and shock following its administration (235).

Less-known methods of decreasing side effects

Other, less-known methods have been explored for decreasing the side effects of chemotherapy; this is through the use of harmless, non-toxic substances. Some of these same substances and regimens may also be used unconventionally to treat cancer or to overcome the effects of chemotherapy after it has been completed.

Most of these methods have not yet been evaluated in randomized clinical trials or other rigorous studies, as they should be if they are to be put into general use. However, they are all without the kind of serious side effects associated with chemotherapy. Thus, even if they turn out not to work, the patient loses little by trying some of them. Patients and their doctors might take note of the following facts:

• Patients undergoing chemotherapy may develop serious vitamin deficiencies, especially of vitamins B1, B2, niacin, folic acid, thiamine, and vitamin K. (On folic acid, see remarks below.) Logically, such vitamins could be replaced in the course of treatment, but rarely are (105).

• Cisplatin causes nerve damage called peripheral neuropathy that looks suspiciously like classic vitamin B12 deprivation. This might be corrected by B12 supplementation. To be fair, one study did not confirm that disruption of vitamin B12 caused this damage (371).

• A large single dose of the B vitamin nicotinamide one hour before taking the drug L-PAM doubled its effectiveness (184). Nicotinamide also "partially reversed" the toxicity of the drug cisplatin in mice (68).

• Vitamin C increased the cell-killing ability of chemotherapy (39). It also blocked heart damage associated with the drugs doxorubicin

(Adriamycin) and interleukin-2 (IL-2). People undergoing high-dose IL-2 treatment suffered a depletion of their bodily reserves of vitamin C that approached frank scurvy. Such deficiencies may contribute to drug toxicity.

It was the observation of two-time Nobel laureate Linus Pauling that: "Vitamin C...controls to a considerable extent the disagreeable side effects of the cytotoxic chemotherapeutic agents, such as nausea and loss of hair, and that benefit seems to add its value to that of the chemotherapeutic agent. We now recommend a high intake of vitamin C, in some cases up to the bowel-tolerance limit [onset of diarrhea, ed.], beginning as early as possible" (296).

In both animal and test-tube experiments, vitamin E reduced the toxicity of the drugs fluorouracil (5-FU), methotrexate, cyclo-phosphamide, and vincristine (358). Since vitamin E and beta carotene are diminished in patients receiving bone marrow transplantation (BMT), German doctors believe that much of the toxicity of BMT is caused by a depletion of vitamins.

"We suggest high-dose supplementation of essential anti-oxidants for patients undergoing BMT," they wrote (72).

A number of cytotoxic drugs were enhanced by vitamin K3 (mena-dione), according to scientists in Taiwan. It also decreased the toxicity of such agents (286).

Do supplements interfere with effectiveness of chemotherapy?
Some doctors are concerned that by reducing toxic side effects one may inadvertently decrease the effectiveness of cytotoxic drugs.

Actually, there is a growing body of literature suggesting that supplementing with nutrients actually *increases* the cytotoxic ability of chemotherapy. Dr. Charles Simone has cited dozens of studies suggesting an enhanced killing of cancer cells by adding vitamins and mineral supplements, especially antioxidants, to chemotherapy.

"Vitamins and minerals do not interfere with the anti-tumor effects of chemotherapy and radiation," Dr. Simone writes. "On the contrary, some vitamins and minerals used in conjunction with chemothera-py...protect normal tissue and potentiate the destruction of cancer cells" (344). For example, he cites studies done at NCI showing that antioxidants protected the hearts of patients receiving doxorubicin (Adriamycin), a cardiotoxic drug, without interfering with its cell-killing ability.

Beta-carotene and other retinoids improved tissue tolerance of animals undergoing both chemotherapy and radiotherapy, with no adverse effect on the tumor-killing ability of these methods. Vitamin E has been shown to have similar effects.

Dangers of folic acid?

On the other hand, the reader should be aware that there is a controversy over the use of the B vitamin folic acid in this regard. The commonly used antimetabolite drug methotrexate works by interfering with folic acid metabolism.

Steve Austin, N.D. warns that "self-administered folic acid supplements are...of concern," to those taking methotrexate, "because they might interfere with the action of the drug. It's unclear," he adds, "whether the small amount of folic acid (usually 400 micrograms) found in multivitamins is enough to be problematic. Discuss it with your oncologist" (26).

On the other hand, a standard text states that "folic acid itself provides poor protection against the toxicity of such drugs as methotrexate" (148). This implies that it does not interfere with it either. *However this is clearly an area that requires consultation with one's doctor.*

A high-intensity supplement formula for people with cancer has been proposed by Brian Leibovitz, Ph.D., editor of the *Journal of Optimal Nutrition*. He gives both a preventative and a therapeutic dose.

Leibovitz's Antioxidant Formula

Antioxidant	Preventative dose	Therapeutic dose
Beta-carotene	15 mg	45 mg
Bioflavonoids	2 grams	8 grams
Coenzyme Q10	100 mg	400 mg
Glutathione	250 mg	1000 mg
N-Acetyl cysteine	600 mg	2400 mg
Non beta-carotene carotenoids (e.g. lycopene)	15 mg	45 mg
Selenium	250 μg*	750 μg*
Vitamin C	2 grams	10 grams
Vitamin E	400 IU	1600 IU

*1 μg or 1 mcg (microgram) = one-millionth of a gram

Most of these supplements are available in larger health food stores or through mail order companies. The carotenoid lycopene is responsible for the red color of the tomato. It is not readily available in health food stores, but is found abundantly in tomato juice and watermelon.

The use of glutamine

In addition, experiments have shown that animals given high doses of the amino acid glutamine were protected against the toxic side effects of high-dose fluorouracil and methotrexate, especially to the digestive tract. Glutamine is essential for the growth of cells in the intestinal lining, a key target of cytotoxic drugs (405).

A randomized, double-blind, prospective clinical study was conducted by doctors at the Harvard-affiliated Brigham and Women's Hospital, Boston, MA (242). They evaluated the metabolic effects of glutamine-supplemented parenteral nutrition in patients who had received bone marrow transplants. They compared hospital charges for the two groups of patients in the trial. The Boston scientists found that the length of hospitalization among patients who were supplemented with glutamine was significantly shorter than in the control group. There was a saving of about one week in the hospital stay per patient.

The incidence of clinical infections was also significantly lower in patients who received glutamine supplementation. Hospital charges were $21,000 less per patient in the glutamine-supplemented group compared to those of patients who received standard therapy. In addition, room and board charges were about $51,000 in the glutamine-supplemented group vs. over $61,000 in the control group (404). Yet the cost of such glutamine supplements is about $5 per day.

Patients may also experience an elevation in mood after taking glutamine (400).

On the other hand, a Dutch study showed no benefits of parenteral glutamine in protecting against the toxicity of chemotherapy (378). And a study from Cambridge also failed to show benefit in treating mouth sores induced by fluorouracil (5-FU) treatments (196).

Glutamine is available in most health food stores or by mail order. A 48 oz. bottle costs about $20.

Herbs

There is some evidence that various herbs, especially those used in Traditional Chinese Medicine (TCM), are also valuable in boosting the immune system and decreasing the side effects of chemotherapy. Some of these are readily available in health food stores or Asian food markets. Medical professionals alone can order most of these from Nuherbs Co., a wholesale distributor in Oakland, CA (1-800-233-4307 or 415-534-HERB). Chinese herbs are best used as directed by a qualified doctor of TCM, since the philosophy behind their use is quite different than that of Western medicine (124).

• Aloe in various forms has shown both preliminary anticancer effects of its own as well as protective effects against the side effects of chemotherapy. In a 1980 study from Madagascar, *aloe vahombe* juice increased the antitumor effects of 5-FU and cyclophosphamide (350). A Russian study has also shown that the juice of ordinary aloe potentiated the effects of the same two drugs (159). Scientists at Memorial Sloan-Kettering have derived novel anticancer agents from emodin, which is found in aloe and many other plants (90,213,214). An aloe extract has also been found to be active against lung cancer cells in the test tube (67). Purified aloe is not known to have any toxicity and can be obtained in drinkable form in most health food stores.

• The herb astragalus (*huang qi*, in Chinese) stimulates the immune system, including that of cancer patients (387). It has also been shown to protect against the ravages of chemotherapy. In mice, it protects the liver and might therefore be used alongside chemotherapy to minimize side effects (402). No toxicity has been shown for this herb. In a Chinese study, a mixture of three herbs including astragalus protected against the toxic side effects of cyclophosphamide (171). A study from the University of Texas concluded that the "reversal of cyclophosphamide-induced immunosuppression" by a partially purified fraction of astragalus "was complete" (71). In TCM, there are reports that astragalus is used in combination with other herbs for an allegedly positive synergistic effect on the immune system (*Boston Globe*, 12/15/86).

• Two Chinese over-the-counter remedies (so-called "kidney tonics") are used in Asia and seem to be of benefit to patients receiving chemotherapy (and/or radiation) for small-cell lung cancer. There were twice as many full or partial regressions in the "tonic" group as among the conventionally treated patients. Median survival was 16 months in the "tonic" group vs. 10 months in the conventional group. In addition, there were four long-term survivors (more than seven years) in the "tonic" group compared to only one such patient in the chemotherapy-alone group (271). The two tonics are *Liu Wei Di Huang* (Six Flavor Tea) and *Jin Gui Shen Qi* (Golden Book Tea). These are available from many Chinese pharmacies or herb supply companies.

Another Chinese preparation said to work well with cyclophosphamide is *Buzhong Yiqi* (or *Bu Zhung Qi Wan*, the "Central Qi Pill"). It increased the activity, while simultaneously decreasing the toxicity, of this widely used drug.

• Scientists were able to significantly decrease the toxicity of platinum-containing drugs (cisplatin and carboplatin) by giving a Japanese "Kampo" herbal mixture to mice with bladder cancer. This mixture is called *Juzen-taiho-to* and it contains astragalus, cinnamon, foxglove, nettle, peony root, angelica, ginseng, licorice, and other herbs.

• The *Lactobacillus* commonly found in milk and cheese (*L. casei*) has been said to "strongly inhibit" the growth of tumors in mice, in combination with the drugs cyclophosphamide, mitomycin, fluorouracil (5-FU), and bleomycin. This significantly prolonged the life span of leukemic mice. This and other beneficial *Lactobacilli* are available in health food stores and are found in cultured milk products, such as yogurt with live cultures. There is no known toxicity to such products.

However, patients taking the drug procarbazine (Matulane) must avoid all foods containing tyramine, including yogurt (see below).

In addition, a number of less-toxic drugs may decrease the side effects and/or increase the effectiveness of chemotherapy. These include aspirin, anticoagulants, dimethyl sulfoxide, hydrazine sulfate, and lithium carbonate. These are discussed in detail in the author's book, *Cancer Therapy*, but should not be taken by people on chemotherapy without medical supervision (271).

In vitro testing

The in vitro drug response assay—in vitro testing, for short (36)—is an individualized way of pre-screening drugs in the laboratory before they are introduced into the patient's body. Using this innovative technique, some doctors claim to get a reasonably good idea in advance of whether a particular agent is likely to kill the cancer cells of a particular patient. If chemotherapy is being contemplated, this approach might save a great deal of time, money, and suffering.

In a British study of 44 patients with lymphatic cancer, the assay correctly predicted seven sensitive and 30 resistant tumors. There were only six false predictions of sensitivity and one false prediction of resistance (34). Other tests have been similarly effective (45,109,392).

In 21 out of 24 cases of multiple myeloma, clinical improvement was said to correspond to a drug's activity in this test. Scientists concluded that in vitro screening should improve the efficacy of subsequent chemotherapy. In melanoma, German doctors concluded that "in vitro drug testing promises to help avoid treatment with ineffective drugs and their associated toxic side effects" (334).

At the present time, about one percent of U.S. patients utilize in vitro testing for chemotherapy. But many doctors will agree to it if the patient brings it to their attention, and some insurance plans pay for it.

In vitro testing does not solve the many problems associated with chemotherapy. But it does hold out the prospect that some people might avoid chemotherapy that won't even cause a response. Others might experience a better outcome by finding the drugs that are best suited to killing their own individual tumor cells.

Sources of in vitro testing

Patients who are contemplating chemotherapy might consider discussing in vitro testing with their doctor. One company that provides such testing is the Weisenthal Cancer Group, headed by Larry Weisenthal, M.D., Ph.D., 15201 Springdale Street, Huntington Beach, CA 92649, (714) 894-0011. They do very extensive and individualized testing, for which they need a source of malignant tissue from the patient's surgeon or oncologist. They generally use three different assays to test cells against 25 to 35 drugs and combinations. Their assessment takes about a week. The test not only points out what is not likely to work, but also which are the most active drugs. According to the company, patients will have a 7.7 fold greater chance of responding to drugs active in this system, as compared to drugs shown to be inactive.

Another company that provides such tests is Oncotech, Inc. Samples of tumor must be sent to the company in a special container for analysis. A patient's physician can contact the company at 1791 Kaiser St., Irvine, CA 92714, (800) 662-6832. They offer two kinds of testing: prognostic markers, and extreme drug resistance.

The reader should bear in mind that in vitro testing does not change the nature or toxicities of the drugs used. Nor does it overcome any of the limitations inherent in cytotoxic agents. Furthermore, it is unclear how often this test results in actually prolonged survival, much less cure. However, if one has decided to take chemotherapy, in vitro testing seems like a logical step to assure the best possible outcome.

Fascinating rhythms

In the early eighteenth century, it was observed that the leaves of the mimosa plant continue to open during daytime hours even when the plant is kept in total darkness. Humans also have such "circadian rhythms." Both cancer cells and normal tissues have varying responses depending on the time of day the drug is given. The toxicity of at least 20 drugs is dependent on the time of day in which the drug is given. This has been clinically demonstrated for fluorouracil, cisplatin, and doxorubicin. Effectiveness can also be dependent on circadian cycles.

This topic should be raised with doctors before patients enter into chemotherapy. Although a full discussion is beyond the purview of this book, we will note, in the words of Dr. DeVita's textbook, that "most clinicians give little thought to the time of day at which a drug is given. In general, patients receive drugs at times that are convenient to the staff administering them," (188) and not when they will be most effective or least toxic.

CHAPTER TEN

Conclusions

A CLOSE LOOK AT CHEMOTHERAPY yields some major surprises. Few would dispute its usefulness in acute lymphocytic leukemia, Hodgkin's disease, testicular and ovarian cancer, and a handful of rare tumors, mainly of childhood. But evidence for the life-prolonging effect in other common malignancies is weak, even for those cancers in which almost certainly it has some marginal success. And proof is simply non-existent for the majority of cancers, especially the advanced carcinomas.

Even for the common cancers in which chemotherapy "works," such as small-cell lung cancer, the actual survival benefit is reckoned in weeks or months, not in years. And during this time, the patient is likely to experience major, even life-threatening side effects from the treatment. Thus, the overall advantage to the patient is moot.

In the adjuvant treatment of breast cancer, the picture is confused. Among premenopausal women, there may be a small statistical advantage in survival rates between those who can and do take the treatment and those who do not. For postmenopausal women, a stronger case can be made for the hormonal agent tamoxifen, although this may be carcinogenic. In advanced breast cancer, there is no compelling evidence that chemotherapy prolongs actual survival.

In colon cancer, there is no evidence of chemotherapy's effectiveness in Dukes' A, B, or D cancer. The situation in Dukes' C is still unclear. But the rush to administer 5-FU plus levamisole, which started in 1990, may backfire. The Harbor-UCLA finding in 1994, showing that adjuvant levamisole taken alone led to a decreased 10-year survival rate, is certainly cause for serious concern.

It is often said that chemotherapy palliates symptoms or improves quality of life. Yet the terms palliation and quality of life are almost never defined, and can mean almost anything. Some people mean by it the promotion of a hopeful attitude—but clearly any substance can be used as a placebo to convey *false* hope. The question is really whether toxic chemotherapy does better than sugar pills.

For most patients, chemotherapy actually represents a serious decrease in their quality of life, due to the rampant toxicity of most of the drugs used. Oncologists have been derelict in not doing reproducible studies to investigate this question. For many patients and their families, chemotherapy is "bottled death," according to the poignant words of Senator Hubert H. Humphrey, just before his own death from bladder cancer (*N.Y. Daily News*, 1/14/78).

One other drawback of chemotherapy is rarely considered. Aggressive chemotherapy reduces the likelihood of benefiting from other promising nontoxic , nutritional, or immunological treatments. One needn't get into a discussion here of the effectiveness of such therapies. (See the author's *Cancer Therapy*.)

But by damaging the bone marrow and various other organs of the body, chemotherapy can diminish the patient's chances of profiting from promising treatments that depend upon enhancing immunity, performance status, and improved functionality.

Chemotherapy also plays a role in the age-old struggle between conventional and unconventional modes of treatment. A leading oncologist once actually argued that despite its record of failure, cytotoxic chemotherapy should still be administered to advanced cancer patients. He stated:

"Nevertheless, chemotherapy serves an extremely valuable role in keeping patients oriented toward proper medical therapy…. Judicious employment and screening of potentially useful drugs may also prevent the spread of cancer quackery….Properly based chemotherapy can serve a useful purpose in preventing improper orientation of the patient" (321).

In such cases, it serves an ideological rather than a medical function. This is a cruel abuse of a patient's rights.

Recommendations

This book is primarily designed to help individuals make decisions about the use of chemotherapy. But I would also like to offer suggestions for what can be done at the level of government and society to help remedy some of the abuses pointed out in this book.

• Require proof of life extension

In clinical trials, "responses" or "disease-free survival" should no longer be accepted as valid criteria for the effectiveness of drugs. Peer-reviewed medical publications should require *proof* of *life extension* and/or well-defined palliative effects, through randomized clinical trials, as the basis for any claims of the effectiveness of cytotoxic agents. Insurers should not pay for toxic chemotherapy that has not been demonstrated, in adequately conducted RCTs, to substantially increase absolute survival of patients and/or to significantly improve their quality of life. Tumor shrinkages, disease-free survival, and other effects unproven to correlate with actual increased survival or real palliation should no longer be accepted as the basis for reimbursement.

• *Include nontoxic alternative in clinical trials*

Nontoxic alternative treatments should be offered as an arm in government-funded chemotherapy trials. Orthodox doctors regard such treatments essentially as placebos (87,228). If, contrary to all expectations, these alternative treatments perform as well as or better than chemotherapy, then it is these alternatives that should be intensively investigated in follow-up studies, rather than the chemotherapy.

Due to the growing popularity of alternative cancer treatments (228), the inclusion of such approaches could spur flagging enrollments in randomized clinical trials. It could also speed the evaluation of alternative treatments, which almost never receive fair, adequate, and speedy evaluations (269). Oncologists should welcome this chance to both resuscitate the whole clinical trial program, and to show their willingness to evaluation less toxic unconventional treatments.

• *Investigate the failure of the "war on cancer"*

The U.S. Congress (as well as similar legislative bodies elsewhere) should initiate an investigation of the failure of the "war on cancer." This should focus on the ways in which the pharmaceutical industry has gained decisive influence over that effort, to the exclusion of other approaches, such as prevention, non-invasive diagnostic techniques, and promising alternative treatment modalities. The major goal should be a sweeping reform of the National Cancer Act of 1971.

• *Include critics in decision-making bodies*

Finally, critics of the cancer establishment should be appointed to leading bodies in the field, including the U.S. National Cancer Advisory Board (NCAB), the President's Cancer Panel, and the various advisory councils of the NIH and the NCI. At every level, there should be a true diversity of views, replacing the "make-work atmosphere" (48) that prevails in so many of these bodies.

The patient's rights

This book offers people with cancer some of the information they need to take a more active role in their choice of treatments. But patients are sometimes confused about what *rights* they have regarding their choices.

Dr. Martin Shapiro of UCLA has told the informative story of a patient of his, a man in his thirties with advanced lung cancer, who had already failed to respond to three different chemotherapeutic regimens.

When he came in to start a fourth one, Shapiro asked him if this was what he really wanted to do.

"Do I have any other choice?" the patient asked. The man was ready to do whatever he thought the doctor wanted, spurred on by stories of the wonders of chemotherapy. "Unduly optimistic publicity helps to create a climate in which patients resign themselves to chemotherapy for conditions in which it does not work," Shapiro concluded (340).

So let me state this clearly: *If you are a sane and sentient adult you have an absolute right to take or refuse any treatment.* You are certainly within your rights to continue chemotherapy, if that is your wish, even if you or your doctor thinks the odds are slim that it will help you. You can also walk away from any cancer therapy situation and nobody can stop you. Here are some other possible choices:

• You may choose the alternative approach. For instance, you may go to a domestic or foreign clinic; work with an alternative doctor or health care practitioner; or procure unconventional treatments that are not necessarily approved of by the government or medical authorities.

• You may choose to enter an experimental protocol sponsored by the NCI, or another such institution. Lists and descriptions of such treatments are available via the computerized PDQ system, or, in the U.S., by calling the NCI's Cancer Information Service at 1-800-4-CANCER.

• Or, you may decide to work with your loved ones and health-care providers to "maximize comfort and function, to sort through the maze of emotional and social problems evoked by the illness, and even to grieve together over the impending death" (340).

You have a right to a copy of your medical records. You can always ask for a second, third, or fourth opinion. You can demand answers to all your questions in a language you can understand. Especially, you can always ask to see proof of the effectiveness of the treatment being offered in terms of actual (not just disease-free) survival and/or improved quality of life.

You always have the right of "informed consent," to be told and understand exactly what is going to be done to you.

And just because it is called *informed consent does not mean that you have to consent,* after you are allegedly informed. At any point, you can refuse. You do not have to be "reasonable" or to live up to anyone else's standards, including your doctor's.

The worst that will happen is that the doctor will get angry. But the doctor should know that if he or she refuses to treat a patient on capricious or unreasonable grounds, this may be actionable behavior.

Medical freedom of choice

Freedom of choice is not a footnote to legal history. It is fundamental to democratic society.

The great political philosopher Thomas Hobbes (1588-1679), although a staunch monarchist, affirmed that even subjects of the Crown had certain rights that could not be trampled on by His Majesty: "Subjects have liberty to defend their own bodies, even against them that lawfully invade them," such as government's agents, and that people "are not bound to hurt themselves" (*Leviathan*, ch. 21).

Many other philosophers and thinkers have upheld this right. But the most ringing statement came from John Stuart Mill (1806-1873). In 1859, Mill predicted that the question of individual freedom was "likely soon to make itself recognized as the vital question of the future." He opposed the "tyranny of the prevailing opinion and feeling" and the repression of minority opinions and behavior. To his everlasting honor, he made "common cause in defense of freedom, with heretics generally."

Mill made no distinction between "right" or "wrong" behavior, when looked at from some other person's perspective. Every person must have freedom of action, "without impediment from our fellow-creatures, so long as what we do does not harm them, even though they should think our conduct foolish, perverse, or wrong."

This point is extremely important. In medicine, for instance, we sometimes hear doctors say that they believe in medical freedom of choice, but only as long as it is "informed choice." Of course it is they, and their surrogates, who will do the informing.

This sort of proviso denies peoples' fundamental right to be "foolish" in other people's eyes. But if such rights are not respected, said Mill, then a society is not free, "whatever may be its form of government."

Mill proclaimed that "the only freedom...is that of pursuing our own good in our own way....Each is the proper guardian of his own health, whether bodily, or mental and spiritual."

"Over himself, over his own body and mind, the individual is sovereign," Mill wrote. Those words should be engraved in stone over the entrance to every cancer center in the world!

Legal opinions

In the United States, there has been a long series of legal opinions upholding the fundamental right to take or refuse medical treatment.

The right of patient autonomy is grounded in a more general "right to privacy," a common-law right that in America was first clearly articulated in a landmark 1890 *Harvard Law Review* (4:193-220) article by Louis Brandeis and Samuel Warren.

Privacy received one of its first expressions in a medical context in a famous 1914 New York case. Judge Benjamin Cardozo (the future Supreme Court justice) utilized this concept in his decision in *Schloendorff v. Society of New York Hospital* [211 N.Y. 125 (1914)]. According to his now-classic formulation:

"Every human being of adult years and sound mind has a right to determine what shall be done with his own body."

When Brandeis himself became a Supreme Court judge, he wrote a famous dissent in *Olmstead v. United States* [(277 U.S. 438 (1928)]:

"The makers of our Constitution undertook to secure conditions favorable to the pursuit of happiness. They recognized the significance of man's spiritual nature, of his feelings, and of his intellect. They knew that only part of the pain, pleasure, and satisfactions of life are to be found in material things. They sought to protect Americans in their beliefs, their thoughts, their emotions and their sensations. They conferred, as against the government, the right to be left alone—the most comprehensive of rights and the right most valued by civilized men."

Commenting on Brandeis's opinion many years later, Judge Warren Burger (the future Chief Justice of the U.S. Supreme Court) wrote:

"[N]othing in this utterance suggests that Justice Brandeis thought an individual possessed these rights only as to sensible beliefs, valid thoughts, reasonable emotions, or well-founded sensations. I suggest that he intended to include a great many foolish, unreasonable, and even absurd ideas which do not conform, such as refusing medical treatment even at great risk" [331 F.2d 1010 (D.C. Cir. 1964)].

So if your doctor argues that your rejection of chemotherapy is "foolish" or "absurd"— so be it. She is entitled to her opinion. But you are still well within your own rights in rejecting it.

In *Andrews v. Ballard* [498 F. Supp. 1038 (1980)], U.S. District Judge Gabrielle McDonald wrote (in a case involving a patient's right to receive acupuncture):

"It is the individual making the decision, and no one else, who lives with the pain and the disease. It is the individual making the decision, and no one else, who must undergo or forgo the treatment. And it is the individual making the decision, and no one else, who, if he or she survives, must live with the results of that decision. One's health is a uniquely personal possession. The decision of how to treat that possession is of a no less personal nature."

What about the right not just to reject chemotherapy, but to receive a treatment that the doctor may disapprove of? In the cancer-related case of *Schneider v. Revici* [817 F. 2d 987 (2nd Cir. 1987)], upheld on appeal, the 2nd Circuit U.S. Court of Appeals held: "We see no reason why a patient should not be allowed to make an informed decision to go outside currently approved medical methods in search of an unconventional treatment."

The same notion was reaffirmed in New York in 1993, when Judge Edward I. Greenfield vacated an order of the New York State Department of Health suspending the medical license of Robert Atkins, M.D. He wrote:

"Patients of course have the right to choose a mode of treatment, or indeed to choose non-treatment, if they are adults capable of arriving at a decision for their own reasons" (cited in *The Cancer Chronicles* 9/93).

But it was California's Chief Justice Rose Bird (herself a cancer survivor) who best summed up the legal perspective:

"Cancer is a disease with potentially fatal consequences; this makes the choice of treatment one of the more important decisions a person may ever make, touching intimately on his being. For this reason, I believe the right to privacy, recognized under both the state and federal constitutions, prevent the state from interfering with a person's choice of treatment on the sole ground that the person has chosen a treatment which the state considers 'ineffective.' " [*People v Privitera*, 23 Cal. 3d at 705 (1979)].

Question your doctor

For the reasons given above, and more, it is extremely important that patients and their families question their doctors and become actively involved in creating a treatment plan.

If there is one lesson to be learned from this book, it is to question your doctor. And the key question to ask is:

"What is the proof that the treatment being offered will either cure, extend actual survival, or increase quality of life?"

Proof. Ask to see the scientific papers and reports on the treatment. If necessary, seek out professional help in interpreting the facts and figures.

You have a moral and legal right to ask for that information. Be on your guard against evasive maneuvers of all kinds. Be especially skeptical of doctors who say, "Our treatment is so new that we have not had a chance to evaluate it yet." They may have said this before to people who took their prior treatment, as well as the one before that. This can be a convenient excuse to obscure a string of failures.

Consider this sage advice from a cancer patient's widow, who wrote to *The Cancer Chronicles* (11/93):

"Question your doctor. Question him every step of the way. The more serious the condition, the more serious the treatment, the more stringent the questioning must be. If you don't have the energy, enlist the help of someone who does....Don't be afraid to fight. Question your doctor, the same way you would a politician, for the two are not dissimilar. If your doctor won't answer the questions, find one that will....There is a party line within the medical system. Question your doctor. Always."

And indeed, some doctors welcome intelligent dialogue, and appreciate the chance to share the complexities of their science with inquisitive patients. Others don't. If a doctor gets angry, condescending, or evasive, it may be time to look for another doctor. Never allow yourself to be hustled. Most likely you pride yourself on being a knowledgeable consumer in the general marketplace. Be an informed medical consumer, as well.

You now have a yardstick by which to measure the effectiveness of cancer treatments. If a drug or regimen has not been proven to cure, significantly prolong actual survival, or improve the quality of life—if it only temporarily shrinks tumors, with a probable loss in well-being—then it is at most entirely experimental and unproven, and should not be represented as anything else. At worst, it could be not just ineffective, but painful, destructive—even fatal.

It may be time to look into other alternative, nutritional, or nontoxic treatments. It is my personal opinion that the best of these treatments are based on more plausible theories and offer more compelling evidence than most chemotherapy; they certainly do far less harm.

Patients and their loved ones are often understandably devastated when they learn that they have cancer. It is an additional blow to learn that chemotherapy is not likely to help, much less cure. But cancer is not a death sentence. It can be a turning point.

The loss of illusions may be the beginning of wisdom.

Cytotoxic Drugs

THE FOLLOWING IS A LIST of the main cytotoxic drugs now being used in the treatment of cancer.

Generic name	Proprietary Name	US Manufacturer
altretamine	Hexalen	US Bioscience
asparaginase	Elspar	Merck
bleomycin sulfate	Blenoxane	Bristol-Myers Squibb
busulfan	Myleran	Burroughs-Wellcome
carboplatin	Paraplatin	Bristol-Myers Squibb
carmustine (BCNU)	BiCNU	Bristol-Myers Squibb
chlorambucil	Leukeran	Burroughs-Wellcome
cisplatin	Platinol	Bristol-Myers Squibb
cyclophosphamide	Cytoxan, Neosar	Bristol-Myers Squibb
cytarabine (ara-C)	Cytosar-U	Upjohn
dacarbazine	DTIC-Dome	Miles
dactinomycin (actinomycin)	Cosmegen	Merck
daunorubicin hydrochloride	Cerubidine	Wyeth-Ayerst
doxorubicin	Adriamycin	Adria
etoposide	VePesid	Bristol-Myers Squibb
fluorouracil (5-FU)	Fluorouracil	Roche
hydroxyurea	Hydrea	Bristol-Myers Squibb
idarubicin	Idamycin	Adria
ifosfamide	IFEX	Bristol-Myers Squibb
lomustine (CCNU)	CeeNU	Bristol-Myers Squibb
mechlorethamine	Mustargen	Merck
melphalan (L-PAM)	Alkeran	Burroughs-Wellcome
mercaptopurine (6-MP)	Purinethol	Burroughs-Wellcome
methotrexate	Methotrexate	Lederle
mitomycin	Mutamycin	Bristol-Myers Squibb
mitotane	Lysodren	Bristol-Myers Squibb
mitoxantrone	Novantrone	Lederle
paclitaxel	Taxol	Bristol-Myers Squibb
plicamycin	Mithracin	Miles
procarbazine	Matulane	Roche
streptozocin	Zanosar	Upjohn
teniposide	Vumon	Bristol-Myers Squibb
thiotepa (TSPA)	Thiotepa	Lederle
thioguanine (6-TG)	Tabloid brand	Burroughs-Wellcome
vinblastine sulfate	Velban	Eli Lilly
vincristine sulfate	Oncovin	Eli Lilly

APPENDIX B

Some Common Protocols

ABV	doxorubicin + bleomycin + vinblastine
BACON	bleomycin + adriamycin + lomustine + vincristine + mechlorethamine
BACOP	bleomycin + doxorubicin + cyclophosphamide + vincristine + prednisone
BOLD	bleomycin + vincristine + lomustine + dacarbazine
CA	cyclophosphamide + doxorubicin
CAMP	cyclophosphamide + doxorubicin + methotrexate + procarbazine
CAP	cyclophosphamide + doxorubicin + cisplatin
CAV	cyclophosphamide + doxorubicin + vincristine
CFPT	cyclophosphamide + fluorouracil + prednisone + tamoxifen
CHOP	cyclophosphamide + doxorubicin + vincristine + prednisone
CHOP-B	cyclophosphamide + doxorubicin + vincristine + prednisone + bleomycin
CISCA	cyclophosphamide + cisplatin+ doxorubicin
CMF	cyclophosphamide + methotrexate + fluorouracil
CMFP	cyclophosphamide + methotrexate + fluorouracil + prednisone
CMFVP	cyclophosphamide + methotrexate + fluorouracil + vincristine + prednisone
COAP	cyclophosphamide + vincristine + cytarabine + prednisone
COMLA	cyclophosphamide + vincristine + methotrexate + leucovorin + cytarabine
COP	cyclophosphamide + vincristine + prednisone
COP-BLAM	cyclophosphamide + vincristine + prednisone + bleomycin + doxorubicin + procarbazine
CVP	cyclophosphamide + vincristine + prednisone
CyVADIC	cyclophosphamide + vincristine + doxorubicin + dacarbazine
FAC	fluorouracil + doxorubicin + cyclophosphamide
FAM	fluorouracil + doxorubicin + mitomycin
Hexa-CAF	altretamine + cyclophosphamide + methotrexate + fluorourcil
ICE	ifosfamide + cyclophosphamide + etoposide
MACC	methotrexate + doxorubicin + cyclophosphamide + lomustine
M-BACOD	bleomycin + doxorubicin + cyclophosphamide + vincristine + dexamethasone + methotrexate + leucovorin
MOPP	mechlorethamine + vincristine + procarbazine + prednisone
MVPP	mechlorethamine + vinblastine + procarbazine + prednisone
ProMACE	prednisone + methotrexate + doxorubicin + cyclophosphamide + etoposide
ProMACE-CytaBOM	cyclophosphamide + doxorubicin + etoposide + prednisone + cytarabine + bleomycin + vincristine + methotrexate + leucovorin
VAC	vincristine + dactinomycin + cyclophosphamide

The Major Drugs

~~~

"Many medicines few cures."
—Benjamin Franklin, *Poor Richard's Almanack*, 1734

The following is a discussion of the major cytotoxic drugs used in the treatment of cancer. They are here arranged according to the subcategories in which they are usually discussed in standard textbooks on cancer. Unless otherwise noted, technical information comes primarily from such books (97,232,396) as well as from the 1995 *Physicians' Desk Reference (PDR)*, which is available in most public libraries.

For consistency's sake, throughout this book we have referred to cytotoxic drugs by their scientific, generic names, even though many of them are far better known by their registered names, by abbreviations, or even by nicknames. Thus, almost everyone refers to a particular new drug as "Taxol," although the scientific name of this compound is paclitaxel. Sometimes drugs have different names in different countries. Altretamine is called Hexalen in the U.S. but Hexastat in Canada. Around the world, cyclophosphamide is actually known by 28 different names! To avoid confusion, in this book we have generally stuck to the generic titles found in the *PDR*.

Also, here as in the above text, we only discuss the *approved cytotoxic drugs*. These include the alkylating agents, antibiotics, antimetabolites, plant-derived agents, platinum-containing agents, as well as miscellaneous antineoplastics. No attempt has been made to discuss drugs used in cancer that do not work by poisoning dividing cells. These would include antineoplastics that alter hormonal balance; biological response modifiers; or drugs that are used in the pharmacological management of adverse reactions. Nor shall we discuss the experimental agents that are currently under development at the National Cancer Institute or elsewhere.

Alkylating Agents

Alkylating agents, as we have noted, were the first class of cytotoxic drugs to be created from mustard gas. These drugs strongly link up with and destroy normal components of the cell, mainly the genetic material (DNA), and are highly toxic.

Cancer cells readily develop resistance to these drugs, and such acquired resistance becomes a vexing clinical problem. That is one reason they often fail and why they are frequently used in combination with other drugs that operate through different mechanisms.

All alkylating agents should be regarded as carcinogenic. Leukemias and other secondary cancers are fairly common among survivors. Up to ten percent of patients who survive ovarian cancer succumb to second cancers caused by these drugs (158). Alkylating agents can also cause serious lung injury (390).

Prolonged use may result in the loss of menstruation in women and a decrease or total inactivation of sperm production in men. Although some individuals have gone on to have children after such chemotherapy, it is not certain that this is desirable, for alkylating agents have been known to cause mutations and fetal malformations in experimental animals. The following are the six main alkylating agents:

Mechlorethamine (Mustargen, nitrogen mustard)

Mechlorethamine hydrochloride was the first non-hormonal drug to be tested against cancer. It was synthesized from mustard gas during World War II. Mechlorethamine is rarely used today as a single agent but is commonly found as part of the MOPP regimen.

Mechlorethamine can have awesome effects on the human body. It is a blistering agent (vesicant), causes severe nausea and vomiting, may cause thrombophlebitis (venous inflammation with clot formation) and sclerosis (hardening) of the veins into which it is administered. Inhalation is dangerous. If it leaks from the needle during administration (extravasation) it can cause severe inflammation. Health workers must put ice packs on the wound for six to twelve hours "to prevent severe, permanent tissue damage" (337).

Mechlorethamine has to be prepared using heavy gloves and biological safety cabinets. If workers inadvertently inhale the powder or its vapors, or come into direct contact with it via skin or mucous membranes, they are themselves in serious medical danger (232).

Melphalan (Alkeran)

This is a synthetic combination of nitrogen mustard and the amino acid, phenylalanine. It was created to selectively target melanoma but didn't work, and is now used to treat other cancers. It is currently used in cancers of the breast, ovaries, and multiple myeloma. Melphalan can be harmful to the liver and kidneys, especially in combination with the immunosuppressant cyclosporine. Tamoxifen may inhibit its activity. Damage to the blood-producing system generally occurs two to three weeks after treatment. Nausea, vomiting, and hair loss are milder than with some other agents, but in the long run, melphalan may cause leukemia. *Dose Range:* three 2-milligram (mg) tablets three times per day. *Wholesale Cost:* $14.58 for 50 2-mg tablets.

Chlorambucil (Leukeran)

Among the slowest acting and least toxic of the alkylating agents, chlorambucil is sometimes used against breast and ovarian cancer, but mainly in chronic lymphocytic leukemia (CLL), macroglobulinemia (a condition seen with multiple myeloma), and one kind of non-Hodgkin's lymphoma. Depression of the immune system is slow and reversible, and nausea is mild or does not occur. It can cause skin rash or hair loss and secondary leukemia. It can also cause sterility in males, liver damage, seizures, protein in the urine, decreased menstruation. Safe use in pregnancy has not been established. *Dose range:* 0.1 to 0.2 mg per kg of body weight per day. *Drug interactions:* None reported. *Wholesale cost:* $6.34 for 50 2-mg tablets.

Busulfan (Myleran)

Used in the treatment of chronic myelocytic leukemia to reduce the number of white blood cells, it is also being tried in patients with acute leukemia. It interferes with the cancer cell's ability to replicate its DNA. It should not be used by pregnant or nursing women. The dose is generally 4 to 8 milligrams per day. It can cause suppression of the bone marrow, scarring of lungs and heart, cataracts, darkened skin color, decreased function of the adrenal gland, skin rash, hair loss, dryness of skin, weakness and jaundice. High doses can lead to general seizures and liver damage. *Wholesale cost:* $3.41 for 25 2-mg tablets.

Cyclophosphamide (Cytoxan)

This is the jack-of-all-trades of chemotherapy. It is generally known as Cytoxan or Neosar (United States), Endoxan (Germany), etc. Cyclophosphamide was introduced clinically in 1958 and soon became the most widely used alkylating agent in the world (204). As of 1995, it had been mentioned in 28,000 medical articles. It causes less gastrointestinal damage than other alkylating agents, even at large doses (79). Cyclophosphamide has become part of regimens for non-Hodgkin's lymphomas, multiple myeloma, breast cancer, and ovarian cancer. It is the "C" in such common regimens as "CMF." It is often used in very high doses in leukemia, but can cause blood deficiencies, hair loss, nausea, and vomiting. It can also cause bleeding in the urinary tract, which may require medical intervention. Patients taking this drug must drink plenty of water and urinate frequently. Other side effects include mouth sores, discoloration of the nails and skin, lung disease and heart damage. *Dose range:* one to five mg per kg body weight per day. *Drug interactions:* It may interact with allopurinol, chloramphenicol, chlorpromazine, steroids, digoxin, methotrexate, blood thinners, succinylcholine, sulfa drugs, certain water pills. *Wholesale cost:* $68.80 for 100 50-mg tablets; $54.33 for one 100-mg vial.

Ifosfamide (IFEX)

This is an look-alike (analog) of cyclophosphamide, first used in the 1970s. In has increasingly been employed in cases of testicular cancer but may be no better than its parent compound (203).

Side effects of the ICE protocol (ifosfamide + carboplatin + etoposide) include mouth sores; inflammation of the intestines; liver toxicity; and damage to hearing, CNS and peripheral nervous system, heart and lung. Up to 94 percent of high-dose patients suffer cardiotoxicity (120).

With ifosfamide, it is said "hallucinations occurred only when the patient's eyes were closed and, in all but one case, were reported as disturbing or frightening" (102). The antidote is a drug, haloperidol, that causes "a statistically significant increase in mammary gland neoplasia" (256). Mesna is given to limit bladder irritation from ifosfamide, although it does not always have the desired effect.

Nitrosoureas

These are a subclass of the alkylating agents. They are highly fat (lipid) soluble and chemically reactive agents. Many related chemicals have been synthesized that differ slightly in their clinical effects. This group has many of the same features as the classic alkylating agents. Common nitrosoureas include:

Carmustine (BiCNU)

Carmustine (BCNU or BiCNU) is used in brain, lymph gland, and plasma cell cancer. The usual dose is 100 to 200 mg per square meter of body surface area, every six weeks. It suppresses bone marrow, causes lowered blood and platelet counts, liver and kidney damage, nausea and vomiting, lung scarring, and burning at the site of injection. It may not be safe for pregnant or nursing women and may interact with dilantin or similar drugs. *Wholesale cost:* $23.19 for one 100-mg vial.

CCNU (Lomustine)

Similar to carmustine and the investigational drug MeCCNU, it is used against lymphomas and brain cancer but is said to be more active against Hodgkin's disease. If regurgitation occurs soon after ingestion, doctors are instructed to examine the patient's vomit for intact capsules. "If these are identified with certainty, the drug should be readministered," say NCI oncologists (395).

Streptozocin (Zanosar)

Although a naturally occurring antibiotic, streptozocin is generally classed with the nitrosoureas. It inhibits DNA synthesis as well as key enzymes involved in the breakdown of sugar (glucose metabolism). Its activity as an alkylating agent is considered weak when compared to other agents. The main use of streptozocin is as a treatment for islet cell tumors of the pancreas, along with fluorouracil. It is also used against adenocarcinomas of the pancreas and metastatic carcinoid tumors. This is a drug of notable toxicity. It causes "severe nausea and vomiting [that] are not very responsive to conventional antiemetics" (395). It is particularly damaging to the beta cells of the pancreas and the kidneys. *Drug interactions:* any drug that affects glucose tolerance or is harmful to the kidneys.

Thiotepa

Thiotepa was a by-product of Germany's World War II mustard gas program. Largely superseded by newer drugs, it is still used in early-stage bladder cancer and occasionally included in combinations for the treatment of breast or ovarian cancer. Thiotepa is relatively mild and causes less nausea and vomiting than some other drugs, but white blood cell damage is common after 10 to 14 days. Side effects may also include pain at the injection site, appetite loss, dizziness, headaches, hives, and asthma-like symptoms. It can also interfere with fertility.

Antimetabolites

An antimetabolite is a molecule designed to closely resemble a necessary, well-tolerated substance, such as a vitamin or an amino acid. Once the look-alike is taken up by the cell, its slight difference puts a monkey wrench into normal cellular functioning. The first antimetabolite was aminopterin, an analog of folic acid. This has been replaced by methotrexate. Methotrexate has been called the most versatile of all chemotherapeutic agents in current clinical use.

Antimetabolites were the product of "rational therapeutics." Unfortunately, like other cytotoxic drugs they cannot distinguish between cancerous and normal tissues and are also taken up by normal fast-growing cells. The result is the poisoning of non-malignant cells and a serious disruption of the normal metabolic needs of the body.

Methotrexate

Methotrexate is a look-alike of folic acid, necessary for the production of healthy red blood cells. It fools cells into absorbing it, where it substitutes itself for the normal vitamin. The result can be disastrous, causing cell destruction and extensive sickness.

Methotrexate is used in the treatment of cancers of the amniotic sac, blood, and the lymph glands. Methotrexate has now been used in dozens of different cancers, in varying doses, including childhood leukemia, osteogenic sarcoma, non-Hodgkin's lymphoma, and chorio-carcinoma. It is also commonly employed in combination for the treatment of breast cancer and is the single standard drug of choice for head and neck cancers. It has also been used in high doses in the treatment of brain cancer or to deliberately suppress the immune system, as in the non-malignant but proliferative skin disease, psoriasis.

Rescue factor

High-dose methotrexate is deadly, but can be used with "rescue," another drug called leucovorin (folinic acid). This prevents patients from dying, summoning them back from what is euphemistically called the "vital frontier." This regimen is abbreviated HDMTX-CF. The whole "package" requires facilities for infusion therapy, hydration, urinary alkalinization, measurement of methotrexate levels, and the detection and aggressive treatment of unpredictable and potentially lethal toxicities.

While rescue supposedly spares people the dangers of high-dose methotrexate, unpredictable and even catastrophic toxicity continues to be seen, even in the hands of experienced investigators.

Methotrexate can cause damage to the immune system and mucous membranes. Depletion of the white blood cells begins about four days after start of treatment. Mouth sores and diarrhea are common, although doctors are supposed to halt the treatment until these problems are resolved. There is disruption of the liver, measured by elevated enzymes. About 25 percent of patients develop liver fibrosis. It also can cause kidney damage in dehydrated patients or when used in high-dose regimens. "Methotrexate pneumonitis," a kind of lung inflammation, is also sometimes seen.

Injections to the brain are associated with toxic effects on the nervous system including acute chemical irritation of membranes lining the brain, paralysis, malfunction of the cranial nerve, seizures, or coma; as well as destruction of the myelin sheath surrounding nerve cells (chronic demyelinating syndrome), resulting in mental deterioration, spastic movements, and coma. "There is no treatment" for these side effects, according to an NCI expert (395).

Proof of high-dose methotrexate's value consists almost entirely of small nonrandomized studies. Optimistic initial reports have generally given way to larger, negative trials. In general, high-dose methotrexate is not believed to be better than standard-dose treatment for the great majority of cancers.

Drug interactions: methotrexate may interact unfavorably with acetazolamide, calcium carbonate, cyclophosphamide, dilantin, magnesium, potassium, probenecid, aspirin, water pills, and tromethamine. *Wholesale cost:* $11.37 for one 50-mg vial.

Fluorouracil (5-FU, Efudex)

Fluorouracil (almost always abbreviated 5-FU) attempts to exploit the cancer cell's perceived affinity for uracil, a normal component of RNA. A poisonous fluorine atom is substituted for hydrogen in the structure of the compound. Two other little used fluoropyrimidines are FUdR and Ftorafur.

Some cancer cells cannot produce enzymes to break down such substances. Theoretically, such tumors may be killed in this way, and 5-FU is widely used to treat cancer of the breast, rectum, stomach, and pancreas, as well as carcinomas of head and neck, esophagus, skin, and anus. In breast cancer, 5-FU is generally combined with cyclophosphamide, vincristine, methotrexate, or doxorubicin. In gastrointestinal (GI) cancer, 5-FU is used either alone or in combination with doxorubicin and mitomycin or semustine. It is now the standard drug, together with levamisole, in the treatment of Dukes' C colon cancer. In head, neck and esophageal cancer, it is used together with cisplatin, in combination with surgery and/or radiation therapy.

Continuous infusions of 5-FU may result in sores in the GI tract, diarrhea, and ulcers. A single large (bolus) injection can suppress the bone marrow. Nausea, vomiting, hair loss, and anorexia are common. White blood cell depression reaches its nadir (low point) one to two weeks from start of therapy. Rashes and darkening of skin are also seen. *Drug interactions:* fluorouracil may interact unfavorably when given with thiazide-type diuretics (water pills). *Wholesale cost:* $13.11 for ten 500-mg ampules for injection.

Cytarabine (Cytosar-U, ara-C)

Cytarabine was isolated in 1951 from an ocean sponge. Similar substances have been isolated from bacterial broths and tested as cytotoxic agents. Cytarabine is said to induce remissions in 50 percent of patients with acute myeloid leukemia (AML). Although patients experience nausea, vomiting, and diarrhea, it is said to be fairly well tolerated. High doses may result in severe suppression of the bone marrow, however. Cytarabine has also been implicated in pancreatitis. When used in high doses, it can cause brain dysfunction, with slurred speech, confusion, coma, and occasional fatalities. *Drug interactions:* cytarabine may interact unfavorably when given in conjunction with digoxin. *Wholesale cost:* $18.50 for one 500-mg vial.

Mercaptopurine (Purinethol or 6-MP)

This drug is mainly used to maintain remissions in acute lymphocytic leukemia (ALL). Side effects may include suppression of the bone marrow and GI tract toxicity. This includes nausea, vomiting, anorexia, and mouth sores. Liver damage occurs in about 30 percent of adult patients. Although jaundice is usually reversible, frank necrosis of the liver can also occur.

Thioguanine (6-TG)

This drug is a structural look-alike of guanine, a substance that is normally found as part of the DNA or RNA. About 30 percent of the drug is absorbed from the gastrointestinal (GI) tract and peak concentrations appear from two to four hours after administration by mouth. It is even faster-acting when taken by intravenous injection. The drug is eventually excreted in the altered form of metabolites.

Thioguanine is mainly used in the treatment of acute nonlymphoblastic leukemia and is used in combination with cytarabine, with or without daunorubicin.

"It is not known to be clinically useful for other neoplasms" (396), but it is being tested broadly in various trials.

Antitumor Antibiotics

These are natural products derived from microbial culture broths of various kinds of *Streptomyces* bacteria. This is the same kind of broth that produces the antibiotic, streptomycin. But antitumor antibiotics are far too toxic to be used against bacterial infections in humans. They kill not just microbes but human cells, both normal and cancerous, by insinuating themselves into the genetic material of the nucleus. Although derived from natural products, the side effects of antitumor antibiotics are similar to those of synthetic drugs and, in some cases, worse.

Some of these agents are probably also carcinogenic. Dactinomycin, for example, has been shown to cause cancer in animals. Two others cause mutations in the standard tests. They probably cause malignancies in patients who live long enough to develop such second cancers. Eight of them are in common use.

Bleomycin sulfate (Blenoxane)

"Bleo" is used in the treatment of squamous cell cancers of the cervix, head and neck, larynx, penis, skin, vulva, as well as cancer of the lymph glands and testicles. The dose range is 25 to 50 units per kg body weight, one to two times weekly. Side effects may include scarring of the lungs (with pneumonia in ten percent of patients), severe allergic reactions, skin rash, itching, fever, chills, vomiting, decreased appetite, weight loss, and pain at the site of the tumor. Other symptoms include hard and/or tender fingertips, nail ridges, discoloration of skin, itchy reddening of skin (pruritic erythema). *Drug interactions:* dilantin or digoxin. *Wholesale cost:* $76.78 for one 15-unit vial.

Daunorubicin hydrochloride (Cerubidine)

This drug is taken up by the liver, metabolized, and distributed throughout the body. It inhibits DNA and RNA synthesis, tearing apart strands of genetic material. It is mainly used in the treatment of acute myeloid leukemia (AML), in which it is said to produce responses in 30 to 50 percent, or in combination with thioguanine, in 60 to 80 percent of cases. Also used in combination with vincristine and prednisone in acute lymphocytic leukemia (ALL), daunorubicin has also demonstrated some activity against solid tumors, but less so than its cousin, doxorubicin. Daunorubicin is highly toxic to white blood cells. It can cause acute and chronic heart damage, with abnormal electrocardiograms, wild heart beats, etc. (384). Congestive heart failure occurs in one to two percent of patients at lower doses, and 12 percent at higher doses. Total heart failure may occur in patients who have received prior radiation to the heart region. Nausea and vomiting from this drug are relatively mild, but may last 24 to 48 hours. Also, reversible hair loss and a bizarre symptom, red urine (which is not caused by internal bleeding) are seen. An accidental escape of the drug from the injection needle (extravasation) can cause severe local irritation and destruction of tissue. *Drug interactions:* none have been reported. *Wholesale cost:* $248.66 for ten 20-mg vials.

Doxorubicin (Adriamycin)

Doxorubicin is another drug that interferes with DNA synthesis. It is broken down by the liver and half is removed from the system in about 30 hours. It has a very broad range of activity against leukemias, sarcomas, and cancers of the breast, bladder, lung, prostate, testis, thyroid, uterus, etc. It forms part of several regimens for leukemias, but has shown no activity against kidney, colorectal cancer, or malignant melanoma. Its side effects are similar to daunorubicin. After 10 to 15 days, there can be a serious depletion of white blood cells. Nausea and vomiting are mild to moderate, but hair loss is nearly universal. Doxorubicin may cause a discoloration of nails and skin. On previously irradiated skin, doxorubicin can cause a "recall" (of previous burns) and the reddening of already healed skin.

Damage to the heart muscle is also seen. One of the most unusual side effects of drugs like this is their ability to cause heart damage. Congestive heart failure also occurs in one to four percent, even at fairly low doses. As the cumulative dose increases, chances of congestive heart failure increase significantly. Doctors are supposed to monitor the heart very carefully when giving this drug. *Drug interactions:* doxorubicin may interact unfavorably when given in conjunction with digoxin or barbiturates. *Wholesale cost:* $18.19 for one 10-mg vial.

Idarubicin (Idamycin)

A close cousin of daunorubicin, idarubicin is said to be eight times more powerful against leukemia in mice. It is also active against Hodgkin's disease and an indolent form of non-Hodgkin's lymphoma. It is employed against advanced breast cancer. In one study there were two complete remissions and 31 partial remissions out of 114 patients (189). By injection, idarubicin is less toxic than either doxorubicin or daunorubicin, causing less severe hair loss, nausea, and vomiting.

Mitoxantrone (Novantrone)

Mitoxantrone strongly inhibits RNA and DNA. It is released very slowly from deep tissues, and ten percent shows up in urine. Mitoxantrone is mainly used in the treatment of ALL, lymphoma, and breast cancer, in which it is somewhat less active than doxorubicin, but also less toxic to the heart and other vital organs. Mitoxantrone is also used in combinations for the treatment of some refractory or relapsed leukemias and lymphomas. Mitoxantrone's main toxicity is to the blood-producing system. Granulocytes are particularly damaged. The worst effects are seen on the twelfth day of treatment. About 30 percent of patients experience nausea and vomiting, and baldness occurs in 10 to 15 percent. One odd effect is that it can turn the patient's fingernails and urine blue.

Mitomycin (Mutamycin)

Mitomycin also interferes with DNA synthesis. It is metabolized in the liver, where it is deactivated within one hour. This drug is said to be active against stomach, pancreatic, breast, head and neck, lung, and cervical cancer. In combination with 5-FU and doxorubicin, mitomycin is widely used against advanced stomach cancer. It is also a second-line treatment against metastatic breast cancer. With mitomycin and 5-FU, combined with radiation, it is said to induce complete remissions in some patients with basiloid carcinomas of the anus. It is also said to be the only agent that undergoes a preferential activation in the low-oxygen environments often found in solid human tumors.

Nausea and vomiting are often seen within a few hours of first treatment and, together with anorexia, can persist for two to three days after treatment. Its main toxic effect, however, is the destruction of white blood cells. This generally occurs after several weeks, but then becomes progressively worse with each new dose. Mitomycin can also cause pneumonia. It has now caused over 200 cases of "hemolytic-uremic syndrome," a reaction that combines severe anemia with acute kidney failure. Sudden internal bleeding in the gastrointestinal tract, as well as blood in urine, in children, is also seen.

Dactinomycin (Actinomycin D, Cosmegen)

This antibiotic was isolated from soil fungi by the celebrated discoverer Selman Waksman (386), but was considered too toxic for human use. Dactinomycin was then found to be active against several types of cancer. It interferes with DNA production and is used, together with radiation, surgery, and other drugs, in the treatment of such rare tumors as nephroblastoma, rhabdomyosarcoma, Ewing's sarcoma, and especially Wilms' tumor. Dactinomycin is said to produce 80 to 90 percent two-year, relapse-free survival in these diseases. It is used in combination with cyclophosphamide and vincristine in the treatment of rhabdomyosarcoma. It is also employed in combinations for treating advanced testicular cancer.

Dactinomycin is said to be as effective as methotrexate in the initial treatment of choriocarcinoma. Dactinomycin can be highly damaging to the blood-producing system, however, starting with the first treatment. Nausea and vomiting occur within a few hours and may be so severe as to force the cessation of treatment. Vomiting can persist between 4 and 20 hours of the treatment. Dactinomycin may also cause diarrhea, mouth sores, and rectal inflammation. In addition, it can cause a severe acne-like condition. Hair loss usually begins after seven days, but is generally reversible.

Plicamycin (Mithracin)

Plicamycin acts by interfering with synthesis of RNA and blocks the action of the parathyroid hormone, responsible for calcium metabolism. It thus has calcium-lowering effects. This drug is so toxic that it has never been systematically evaluated. Plicamycin has been used primarily to treat disseminated germ cell tumors of the testis; now it is used even less. Plicamycin is also used in small doses to treat excessive amounts of calcium in the blood, a condition called severe hypercalcemia. It can cause major damage to the bone marrow, liver, and kidneys, as well as coagulation defects; white and red blood cell depletion; severe elevation of liver enzymes; and protein in the urine (a sign of kidney damage). One skin's may become thick, coarse and red.

Platinum Analogs

One NCI chemotherapist has called the platinum-containing compounds "the most important group of agents now in use for cancer treatment" (316). This class is often said to be "curative" for both testicular and ovarian cancer and also plays a central role in the treatment of lung, head and neck, and bladder cancers. There are two such agents in general use: cisplatin (Platinol) and carboplatin (Paraplatin).

Cisplatin (Platinol)

Cisplatin binds to DNA and produces lesions ("crosslinks" and "adducts") within the genetic material. Its cytotoxic effects are supposedly derived from these effects on genetic material. In the presence of these toxic metals, the DNA's three-dimensional shape changes as it is forced to accommodate the rigid platinum molecule.

Cancers react in very different ways to the two platinum compounds, and in addition there are a great deal of individual reactions among patients: even within a given type of cancers, different tumors differ greatly in their sensitivity to the drug.

The toxicity of cisplatin can be staggering. This may include kidney malfunction, nausea and vomiting, nerve damage, impairment of both sight and hearing, suppression of the bone marrow, and occasionally seizures. The most troublesome of all these are the kidney, nerve and ear damage, for these results are cumulative and, at best, only partially reversible.

Cisplatin can also, more rarely, trigger cardiac arrhythmia, damage to brain tissue, glucose intolerance, and inflammation of the pancreas (pancreatitis) and, if the patient survives, leukemia.

The dose-limiting toxicity (i.e., the reason that the treatment must finally be scaled back) has generally been kidney damage. Peripheral neuropathy is said to resemble the toxicity seen with classic vitamin B12 deprivation. But little research has explored this intriguing finding and there is no indication that vitamin B12 has ever actually been given to patients in an attempt to limit toxicity.

Carboplatin (Paraplatin)

Carboplatin is said to be significantly less toxic than its cousin, cisplatin. It is used in the treatment of ovary, cervix, small-cell lung, head and neck, bladder, testis, mesothelioma, and brain cancers. The side effects, however, are similar to those of cisplatin, although somewhat less severe. These may include low blood counts, nerve damage, hearing loss, toxicity to kidneys, nausea, vomiting, loss of appetite, diarrhea, constipation, mouth sores, and an altered sense of taste.

Miscellaneous Agents

Altretamine (Hexamethylmelamine, Hexalen)

This is a structurally unique agent with an uncertain mechanism of action. It is sometimes used against breast cancer, lymphomas, and small-cell lung cancer. It is frequently used as a second-line therapy for ovarian cancer. It may produce nausea and vomiting as its dose-limiting toxicity. It can lead to mood alterations, hallucinations, and nerve damage. Yet, according to NCI's Dr. Chabner, the side effects of these drugs are "relatively mild" (66).

Dacarbazine (DTIC-Dome)

Synthesized as an antimetabolite but failing in that capacity, dacarbazine is sometimes recategorized as an alkylating agent. Dacarbazine is now believed to be the most active single agent for the treatment of metastatic melanoma. About 25 percent of such patients have remissions. It is also a component in the ABVD regimen for Hodgkin's disease. It causes a 15 percent response rate in soft-tissue sarcomas of adults, usually in combination with doxorubicin.

This drug causes the most severe nausea and vomiting of all cytotoxic drugs, one to three hours after the first injection. With no effective countermeasures, unbearable nausea may lead patients to refuse further therapy. It may also cause fever and malaise as well as muscle aches and pains. Diarrhea is common. Patients are not allowed out in the sun for a day or so, because of the possibility of severe burning after taking this drug. It also causes facial flushing, loss of sensation, and lightheadedness. At least 15 patients have died of acute liver poisoning after taking this drug (65).

Hydroxyurea (Hydrea)

This is used for the treatment of certain blood cancers, cancer of the head and neck, and of the ovaries. Its mechanism of action is basically unknown. The dose range is 20 to 80 mg per kg body weight per day. Side effects of hydroxyurea include suppression of the bone marrow's ability to produce blood cells and platelets, irritation of the mouth, nausea, vomiting, diarrhea, constipation, skin rash, a burning sensation upon urination, loss of hair, drowsiness, headache, seizures, and decreased kidney function. *Drug interactions:* none reported. *Wholesale cost:* $42.76 for 100 500-mg capsules.

Mitotane (Lysodren)

Also called o,p'-DDD, this drug is closely related to the banned insecticide DDT. Mitotane has one primary use in cancer: to block the synthesis of the adrenocortical hormone in both normal and malignant cells. It is mainly used in the palliative treatment of inoperable cancer of the adrenal gland.

About 40 percent is absorbed when it is taken by mouth. It is then slowly degraded by the liver and kidneys and is distributed to the body's fat reserves. Mitotane has a very long half-life in the body, and can in fact be measured there up to nine weeks after administration.

Doctors should probably decrease the dosage in the presence of significant liver or kidney impairment.

Drug interactions: Mitotane increases the metabolism of such drugs as barbiturates, warfarin, and phenytoin (an anticonvulsant). When it is administered along with other central nervous system depressants, it can exacerbate their effects. Toxicity includes gastrointestinal disturbances, visual disturbances, lethargy, and depression. A maculopapular rash (e.g., hives) occurs in 15 percent of the patients given mitotane.

Procarbazine (Matulane)

This is frequently used in the treatment of brain cancer and Hodgkin's disease, although its mechanism of action is poorly understood. In animal experiments, it is a potent immunosuppressant and highly teratogenic (i.e., can cause a malformed fetus). It causes cancer in monkeys. Patients receiving the MOPP regimen (that includes this drug) have an increased incidence of both solid tumors and leukemias. Procarbazine is believed to be the leading carcinogen in this combination. When given orally to humans, its immediate effects include a moderate nausea and a decrease in appetite, as well as blood problems (leukopenia and thrombocytopenia). It also is a mild hypnotic.

Patients receiving procarbazine are warned to avoid foods such as wine, bananas, yogurt and ripe cheese, that contain tyramine, which may trigger a "hypertensive crisis." It also acts similarly to the drug Antabuse, causing sweating, flushing, and headaches when taken with alcohol. Given intravenously, it may cause confusion or coma. The "clinical benefit of this schedule is uncertain" (15). Procarbazine frequently causes lung problems and a maculopapular rash (e.g., hives). According to NCI's Dr. Chabner, however, "the development of a rash is not cause for withdrawal of procarbazine" (66).

Asparaginase (Elspar)

To most people, the nutritional treatment of cancer means giving the body the food and supplements it needs to fight the disease and normalize the body's metabolism. To chemotherapists, such as Dr. Chabner, however, it has a quite different meaning. For him and his colleagues, nutritional therapy of cancer is directed at identifying the differences between the host and malignant cells that might be exploited in treatment. These attempts, he adds, have largely been unsuccessful "because of difficulties in producing a deficiency state by dietary means" (66).

The one exception has been the use of an enzyme called asparaginase. In a celebrated experiment in 1953, a scientist found that the serum of guinea pigs had an antileukemic effect when injected into mice (210). Asparaginase is still used in the treatment of ALL.

The drug causes a possible allergic reaction. Anaphylactic shock may occur with the first dose, and hives, swelling of the voice box, spasms of the lungs, and low blood pressure with subsequent treatments. Up to 50 percent of children experience allergic reactions. The drug's inhibition of protein synthesis may lead to clotting difficulties, hemorrhages, etc. In 25 percent of the children it causes brain dysfunction, confusion, stupor, and coma.

Plant-Derived Agents

A number of cytotoxic drugs are derived from plants. These include the vinca alkaloids, epipodophyllotoxins, and paclitaxel (Taxol). Some are traditional herbal drugs, like the Native American Mayapple. Others are known poisons. Natural or not, most of these drugs, in their purified form at least, are of limited use because of extreme toxicity.

Vincristine sulfate (Oncovin)

The periwinkle (*Vinca rosea*) is a creeping plant that grows wild in Europe and is cultivated there and in the U.S. It has long been used in folk medicine as an astringent, sedative, and diarrhea remedy. A periwinkle extract was tested as an oral remedy for low blood sugar in 1949. It failed that test but did manage to accidentally suppress the bone marrow, where white blood cells are produced. Vincristine, an alkaloid salt of the periwinkle, was introduced in 1958.

Vincristine is used to treat acute lymphocytic leukemia (ALL), Hodgkin's disease, non-Hodgkin's lymphoma, Wilms' tumor, Ewing's sarcoma, and childhood rhabdomyosarcoma. In combination with cyclophosphamide, it is said to produce high remission rates in neuroblastoma. It is also used in combinations for SCLC, breast cancer, and multiple myeloma.

Vincristine increases the accumulation of methotrexate in cancer cells, especially in acute myeloblastic and lymphocytic leukemia. The poison derived from this product of natural origin is as dangerous as many entirely synthetic chemicals. It is very irritating and must be given intravenously. If the drug leaks out during administration (extravasation), it can cause significant skin damage. Vincristine can also cause nerve damage, including the loss of various sensations and even whole senses. Sometimes it causes palsy or severe constipation, abdominal pains, and bowel obstruction.

Vinblastine sulfate (Velban)

Also derived from the periwinkle plant, vinblastine was introduced in 1961. It has a destructive effect on both proteins and DNA. Vinblastine is used to treat advanced Hodgkin's disease and testicular cancer. It is usually used in combination with doxorubicin, bleomycin, and dacarbazine in various regimens. It is also given to relieve the symptoms of breast cancer and three diseases: the rare mycosis fungoides and choriocarcinoma, as well as the once-rare Kaposi's sarcoma. Damage to white blood cells is common within five to ten days. Nausea is relatively mild, but constipation and mouth sores are frequently seen. Mild and reversible hair loss, rashes and sensitivity to light are also seen. Continuous infusions can lead to hepatitis. Extravasation of vinblastine is particularly dangerous. If it occurs, injections must be stopped immediately.

Etoposide (VePesid)

This is an extract of the mandrake, or Mayapple, plant (*Podophyllum peltatum*). It was used for centuries by Native Americans as a cathartic and to treat parasites and venereal warts. (They also occasionally used it to commit suicide.) In the 1940s, one constituent was found to stop cell growth. Early drugs were extremely toxic. However, eventually etoposide was found to be usable in treating non-Hodgkin's lymphoma, germ cell malignancies, leukemias, and small-cell lung cancer.

Etoposide is currently used in the treatment of testicular cancer and non-Hodgkin's lymphoma. It is the single most active standard agent used against NSCLC. It is prominently used as part of the "ICE" regimen against Ewing's sarcoma and many other late-stage cancers. It may cause a depletion of white blood cells and about 30 percent of patients experience nausea and vomiting. Another two percent experience severe allergic reactions. There has been critical, but reversible, nerve damage in patients receiving very high doses.

Teniposide (Vumon, VM-26)

Teniposide is closely related to the above drug, etoposide. They are both technically called epipodophyllotoxins, i.e., drugs derived from the mandrake plant. Like etoposide, teniposide is used against a wide variety of cancers, including both Hodgkin's and non-Hodgkin's lymphomas, germ cell malignancies, leukemias, bladder, and small-cell lung cancers. It is also used in neuroblastoma, but as an off-label use (232). Both are said to possess "a number of basic similarities in their pharmacological characteristics, toxicities, and spectrum of antineoplastic action" (66).

Paclitaxel (Taxol)

Paclitaxel (Taxol) is an alkaloid isolated from the bark of the Western yew tree (*Taxus brevifolia*). In the 1960s a yew extract was reported to have cytotoxic activity. In 1971, Taxol was identified as the active ingredient and by 1979 was shown to stop the division of cells by interfering with the shape and the functionality of tiny intracellular structures called microtubules. Technically speaking, Taxol actually increases the stability of these microtubules, making them rigid. This rigidity interferes with normal cell division.

At first, Taxol was mainly of interest to scientists investigating the structure of such microtubules. Then, in the mid-1980s, scientists began to seriously study its interaction with cancer. It was found to have a marked cytotoxic effect on prostatic cancer cells. Scientists found that it exerted its effects even at low concentrations.

Taxol is considered the most important new agent of the last decade. Excitement derives from its unusual mechanism of action and its ability to cause "responses" in some tumors that no longer respond to conventional chemotherapy. Response rates in refractory ovarian cancer are said to range between 21 and 40 percent. Phase III studies are underway to assess its role in that disease. "Significant activity" has also been claimed in metastatic breast cancer patients (183). It is not yet clear if this activity will translate into a survival advantage.

In an early trial at the Albert Einstein Cancer Center in New York City, Taxol was administered to 26 patients. Three other drugs were first administered to these patients in an attempt at preventing the kind of hypersensitivity (allergic) reactions commonly seen in earlier studies of the yew-derived agent. 40 percent suffered nerve damage, which kept the doctors from giving them more of the drug.

Many patients also showed a significant depletion of neutrophils. This effect tended to be of brief duration. Partial responses that lasted more than three months were seen in 4 of the 12 melanoma patients treated with Taxol (391).

When it was given as an IV drip every three weeks at Johns Hopkins, doctors saw significant damage to the white blood cells (thrombocytes). Nerve damage was also "frequently seen at the highest dosage," with numbness and abnormal sensations in the hands and feet. In some cases, the Baltimore doctors said, "this appeared to be a cumulative effect" (329).

Total loss of hair was common. Other toxic effects included nausea and vomiting; inflammation of the mucous membranes (mucositis); muscle pains (myalgias); and inflammation of veins (phlebitis). At first, they frequently saw heart and lung toxicity but claimed this could be ameliorated by prolonging the infusions and pre-treating the patients with other drugs, such as corticosteroids and antihistamines.

Rapid heart beat occurred in a high proportion of patients, including 29 percent of those with ovarian cancer. Even more serious heart disturbances were experienced by 7 of 140 patients. In 1991, Johns Hopkins' doctors said they wanted "to alert investigators to the potential for these adverse effects. Investigators should continue to maintain a high degree of caution" while using Taxol (47).

Other side effects included nerve damage, hair loss, muscle pains, severe joint pains, nausea, vomiting, diarrhea, and an acute lung reaction—all caused by this "natural" treatment.

The treatment also destroyed white blood cells. This was associated with septic infection in three patients, two of whom died. Other adverse effects included muscle and joint pains, hair loss, diarrhea, nausea, vomiting, and nerve damage. There were also several cases of heart and central nervous system toxicity. The Johns Hopkins' scientists conclusion was that Taxol "is an active agent in drug-refractory ovarian cancer." They further concluded that it should be tried, together with conventional drugs, "in previously untreated patients with advanced ovarian cancer" (113,253).

In early 1993, Taxol was approved by the FDA for the treatment of ovarian cancer and, in April 1994, for breast cancer. Favorable publicity about Taxol initially produced near-hysteria among people trying to get the drug. This in turn led to pressures to harvest the last of the Western yews and to conflicts between cancer advocates and environmentalists. With recent reports that the drug has been oversold, enthusiasm has waned somewhat. It also turns out that the shortage of the drug was greatly exaggerated.

Synthetic form

Rhone-Poulenc, a giant French pharmaceutical company, has developed a synthetic form of paclitaxel, called Taxotere, from European yew trees. This is said to be less toxic and more effective.

It is now considered "a potentially important chemotherapeutic agent for the treatment of cancer," according to scientists at Jerusalem's Hadassah Medical School of Hebrew University and the Albert Einstein School of Medicine in New York. Taxotere is of special interest not only because it is active against cancer, say researchers, but also because the chemical from which it is derived has been isolated from yew (*Taxus baccata*) needles. Unlike bark, the needles can regenerate themselves. Taxotere works like Taxol, but is said to be 2.5-fold more potent than the original drug in several cancer cell lines and at least five times more potent in Taxol-resistant cells.

However, in late 1994, an FDA advisory panel turned down the French company's application for marketing, saying Taxotere had still not been tested sufficiently. Rhone-Poulenc studied 135 women with advanced breast cancer. According to the data presented to the FDA, about 41 percent responded to Taxotere, and it stopped the cancer's progression for about 16 to 19 weeks. Median survival was about 11 months.

In NSCLC, they studied 88 advanced patients: there were responses in 17 percent of the cases and median survival was 9 months. However, the company claimed that 38 percent of patients survived one year, and 20 patients lived 18 months or more. Side effects included serious fluid retention in the limbs and lungs and depletion of immune cells in about half the 931 patients who tested Taxotere for safety. Four percent of the patients died from the drug itself (282).

References

1. Aapro, MS. Review of experience with ondansetron and granisetron. Ann Oncol 1993;4S:9-14.
2. Abel, U and Becker, N. Geographical clusters and common patterns in cancer mortality of the Federal Republic of Germany. Arch Environ Health 1987;42:51-57.
3. Abel, U. Chemotherapy of advanced epithelial cancer: a critical survey. Stuttgart: Hippokrates Verlag, 1990.
4. Abel, U. Chemotherapy of advanced epithelial cancer: a critical review. Biomedicine & Pharmacotherapy 1992;46:439-452.
5. Abel, U. Personal communication, 5/16/94.
6. Adair, FE and Bagg, HJ. Experimental and clinical studies on treatment of cancer by dichloroethylsulfide (mustard gas). Ann Surg 1931;93:190.
7. Agency for Health Care Policy and Research. The national bill for diseases treated in US hospitals: HHS, Rockville, MD. Feb. 1994.
8. A'Hern, RP, et al. Does chemotherapy improve survival in advanced breast cancer? A statistical overview. Br J Cancer 1988;57:615-618.
9. Alberto, P, et al. Chemotherapy of small cell carcinoma of the lung: comparison of cyclic alternative combinations with simultaneous combinations of four or seven agents. Eur J Cancer Clin Oncol 1981;17:1027-1033.
10. American Cancer Society. Cancer facts and figures–1994. Atlanta: ACS, 1994.
11. American Cancer Society. Cancer facts and figures–1995. Atlanta: ACS, 1995.
12. Anderson, C. How not to publicize a misconduct finding. Science 1994;263:1679.
13. Anderson, JR and Korzun, AH. Chemotherapy vs. hormonal therapy in advanced breast cancer [correspondence]. NEJM 1986;315:1092.
14. Angier, N. The lab as battlefield. New York Times Book Review, 3/24/91.
15. Anon. The reporting of unsuccessful cases. Boston Med Surg J 1909;263-264.
16. Anon. Chemotherapy danger cited. Los Angeles Times, 3/14/88.
17. Anon. Ein gnadenloses zuviel an therapie: teil zweifel an den chemischen waffen. Der Spiegel 1987;26:128.
18. Anon. Nausea from chemotherapy eased. Los Angeles Times, 2/4/91.
19. Anon. Gilead Sciences presents highly statistically significant efficacy data. News release. Jan. 31, 1995.
20. Anon. Side glance: laboratory-bred mice. JNCI 1995;87:248.
21. Anon. Search begins for new NCI director; committee named. JNCI 1995;87:253-254.
22. Anon. A mother loses life so twins can be born. New York Times, 2/13/95.
23. Anon. Targeted leukemia treatment meets with success in mice. New York Times, 2/10/95.
24. Antman, K, et al. A phase II study of high-dose cyclophosphamide, thiotepa, and carboplatin with autologous marrow support in women with measurable advanced breast cancer responding to standard-dose therapy. JCO 1992;10:102-110.

REFERENCES

25. Arriaganda, R, et al. Prognosis value of initial chemotherapy doses in limited small cell lung cancer. In: Arriaganda, R. [ed.] Treatment modalities in lung cancer. Basel: Karger, 1988;194-198.

26. Austin, SN and Hitchcock, C. Breast cancer: what you should know (but may not be told) about prevention, diagnosis and treatment. Rocklin, CA: Prima, 1994.

27. Bailar, JC III. Mammography: a contrary view. Ann Inter Med 1976;84:77-84.

28. Bailar, JC III and Smith, E. Progress against cancer? NEJM 1986;314:1226-1232.

29. Baum, M, et al. Measurement of quality of life in advanced breast cancer. Acta Oncol 1990;29:391-395.

30. Beatson, GT. Treatment of cancer of the breast by oophorectomy and thyroid extract. Br Med J 1901;2:1145-1151.

31. Bennett, JT and DiLorenzo, TJ. Unhealthy charities: hazardous to your health and wealth. NY: Basic Books,1994.

32. Berkow, R [ed.] Merck manual of diagnosis and therapy. Rahway: Merck, 1992.

33. Berman, B and Larson, D. [eds.] Alternative medicine: expanding medical horizons. Washington, DC: Gov't. Printing Office (NIH No. 94-066), 1994.

34. Bird, MC, et al. Long-term comparison of results of a drug sensitivity assay in vitro with patient response in lymphatic neoplasms. Cancer 1988;61:1104-1109.

35. Birkhead, BG and Jackson, RRP. Randomized trials: a perspective. In: Slavin and Staquet, 1986.

36. Bissery, MC and Chabot, GG. [History and new development of screening and evaluation methods of anti-cancer drugs used in vivo and in vitro.] Bull Cancer (Paris) 1991;78:587-602.

37. Black, Sir D. The paradox of medical care. J R Coll Physicians Lond 1979;13:57.

38. Bloch, RA. An open letter to cancer center directors. JNCI 1995;87:143.

39. Block, G. Vitamin C and cancer prevention: the epidemiological evidence. Amer J Clin Nutr 1991;53:270S-282S.

40. Bobst, E. Bobst: autobiography of a pharmaceutical pioneer. NY: McKay, 1973.

41. Bonadonna, G. Combination chemotherapy as an adjuvant treatment in operable breast cancer. NEJM 294:405-410, 1976.

42. Bonadonna, G, et al. The CMF program for operable breast cancer with positive axillary nodes: update analysis on the disease-free interval, site of relapse and drug tolerance. Cancer 1977;39:2904-2915.

43. Bonadonna, G, et al. Adjuvant chemotherapy trials in resectable breast cancer carried out in Milan. 4th Intl. Conf. on Adjuvant Therapy of Cancer: Abstr. 34. 1984.

44. Bonadonna, G. Evolving concepts in the systemic adjuvant treatment of breast cancer. Cancer Res 1992;52:2127-2137.

45. Bosanquet, AG. Correlations between therapeutic response of leukaemias and in-vitro drug-sensitivity assay. Lancet 1991;337:711-714.

46. Boyse, M, et al. Adjuvant therapy of colorectal cancer. JAMA 1988;259:3571-3578.

47. Brandwein, MS, et al. Fatal pulmonary lipid embolism associated with taxol therapy. Mt Sinai J Med 1988;55:187-189.

48. Braverman, A. Medical oncology in the 1990s. Lancet 1991;337:901-902.

49. Brescia, FJ. Specialized care of the terminally ill. In: DeVita, 1993;2501-2508.

50. Bristol-Myers Squibb. Uncompromising science [ad]. Science 1995;267:1047.

51. Bross, ID, et al. Is Toxicity really necessary? I. The question. Cancer 1966;19: 1780-1784.

52. Bross, ID, et al. Is toxicity really necessary? II. Sources and analysis of data. Cancer 1966;19:1785-1795.

53. Bross, ID, et al. Is Toxicity really necessary? III. Theoretical aspects. Cancer 1966;19:1796-1804.

54. Bross, ID. Statistical testing of a deep mathematical model for human breast cancer. Journal of Chronic Diseases 1968;21:493-506.

55. Bross, ID. Fifty years of folly and fraud in the name of science. Buffalo, NY: Biomedical Metatechnology Press, 1994.

56. Bross, I. The NSABP trials [letter]. NEJM 1994;331:809.

57. Brower, M, et al. Treatment of extensive stage small cell bronchogenic carcinoma. Am J Med 1983;75:993-1000.

58. Brunner, KW, et al. Adjuvant chemotherapy with cyclophosphamide (NSC-26271) for radically resected bronchogenic carcinoma: A nine year follow-up. In: Muggia, F. and Rozencweig, M. [eds.] Lung cancer: progress in therapeutic research, NY: Raven Press, 1979:411-420.

59. Cairnross, JG and Macdonald, DR. Central nervous system staging. In: Wittes, 1991.

60. Cairns, J. The treatment of diseases and the war against cancer. Sci Am 1985; 253:51-59.

61. Carmichael, J. Cancer chemotherapy: identifying novel anti-cancer drugs. BMJ 1994;308:1288-1290.

62. Carroll, KB, et al. A comparison between a single agent short course chemo-therapy regime and a quadruple prolonged course regime for small cell bronchogenic carcinoma of limited extent. Br J Dis Chest 1983;79:171-178.

63. Carter, R. The gentle legions. NY: Doubleday, 1961.

64. Cavelli, F, et al. Gleichzeitige oder sequentielle hormono-chemotherapie sowie vergleich verschiedener polychemotherapien in der behandlung des metas-tasierenden mammakarzinoms. Schweiz med Wschr 1982;112:774-783.

65. Ceci, G, et al. Fatal hepatic vascular toxicity of DTIC. Cancer 1988;61:1988-1991.

66. Chabner, BA. Anti-cancer drugs. In: DeVita, 1993:325-417.

67. Chan, TC, et al. Selective inhibition of the growth of ras-transformed human bronchial epithelial cells by emodin, a protein-tyrosine kinase inhibitor. Biochem Biophys Res Commun 1993;193:1152-1158.

68. Chen, G and Pan, QC. Potentiation of the anti-tumor activity of cisplatin in mice by 3-aminobenzamide and nicotinamide. Cancer Chemother Pharmacol 1988;22:303-307.

69. Chlebowski, RT, et al. Survival of patients with metastatic breast cancer treated with either combination or sequential chemotherapy. A western cancer study group project. Cancer Res 1979;39:4503-4506.

70. Chlebowski, RT, et al. Late mortality and levamisole adjuvant therapy in colorectal cancer. Brit J Cancer 1994;69:1094-1097.

71. Chu, DT, et al. Immunotherapy with Chinese medicinal herbs. II. Reversal of cyclophosphamide-induced immune suppression by administration of fractionated astragalus membranaceus in vivo. J Clin Lab Immunol 1988;25:125-129.

72. Clemens, MR, et al. Decreased essential antioxidants and increased lipid hyperperoxides following high-dose radiochemotherapy. Free Radic Res Commun 1989;7:227-232.

73. Coates, A. On the receiving end: patient perception on the side-effects of cancer chemotherapy. Eur J Cancer Clin Oncol 1983;19:203-208.

74. Coates, A, et al. Improving the quality of life during chemotherapy for advanced breast cancer. NEJM 1987;317:1490-1495.

75. Cohen, AM, et al. Colon cancer. In: DeVita, 1993;929-977.

76. Cohen, CJ, et al. Improved therapy with cisplatin regimens for patients with ovarian carcinoma (FIGO stages III and IV) as measured by surgical end-staging (second look operation). Am J Obstet Gynecol 1987;5:955-967.

77. Cohen, MH, et al. Intensive chemotherapy of small cell broncogenic carcinoma. Cancer Treat Rep 1977;61:349-354.

78. Cohen, V. Should the patient be told? Washington Post. 4/23/86.

79. Colvin, OM and Chabner, BA. Alkylating agents. In: Chabner, BA and Collins, JM [eds.] Cancer chemotherapy: principles and practice. Philadelphia: J.B. Lippincott, 1990: 276-313.

80. Consensus-development-konferenz zur therapie des metastasierten mammakarzinoms. Leitlinien zur palliativen behandlung. Munch Med Wschr 1988;130:93-102.

81. Cooke, CE and Mehra, IV. Oral ondansetron for preventing nausea and vomiting. Am J Hosp Pharm 1994;51:762-771.

82. Cooley, CH. Human nature and the social order. NY: Scribner's, 1922:352-353.

83. Cormier, Y, et al. Benefits of polychemotherapy in advanced non-small cell bronchogenic carcinoma. Cancer 1982;50:845-849.

84. Coulter, HL. The controlled clinical trial. Washington, DC: Center for Empirical Medicine, 1991.

85. Coulter, HL. Divided legacy. Washington, DC: Center for Emp. Medicine, 1994.

86. Crewdson, J. Head of federal cancer institute plans to resign. Chi. Trib. 12/22/94.

87. Curt, GA. Unsound methods of cancer management. In: DeVita, 1993;2734-2747.

88. Cutuli, BF, et al. [Cancer of the breast after Hodgkin's disease. Analysis of 6 cases (letter)]. Presse Medicale-Paris 1993;22:1928-1929.

89. Daniels, JR. Chemotherapy of small cell carcinoma of the lung: A randomized comparison of alternating and sequential combination chemotherapy programs. JCO 1984;2:1192-1199.

90. Darzynkiewicz, Z, et al. Effect of derivatives of chrysophanol, a new type of potential anti-tumor agents of anthraquinone family, on growth and cell cycle of L1210 leukemic cells. Cancer Lett 1989;46:181-187.

91. Davidson, RA. Source of funding and outcome of clinical trials. J Gen Intern Med 1986;1:155-158.

92. Davis, S, et al. Single agent and combination chemotherapy for extensive non-small cell carcinoma of the lung. Cancer Treat Rep 1980;64:685-688.

93. Davis, S, et al. Combination cyclophosphamide, doxorubicin and cisplatin (CAP) chemotherapy for extensive non-small cell carcinomas of the lung. Cancer Treat Rep 1981;65:955-958.

94. Demark-Wahnefried, W, et al. Why women gain weight with adjuvant chemotherapy for breast cancer [review]. JCO 1993;11:1418-1429.

95. DeVita, VT, Jr., Progress in cancer management. Cancer 1983;51:2401-2409.

96. DeVita, VT, Jr., et al. Hodgkin's Disease. In: DeVita, 1993:1819-1858.

97. DeVita, VT, Jr., et al. [eds.] Cancer: principles & practice of oncology. Philadelphia: J.B. Lippincott, 1993.

98. Dexeus, FH, et al. Chemotherapy for advanced squamous carcinoma of the male external genital tract and urethra. In: Johnson, DE, et al. [eds.] Systemic therapy for genitourinary cancers. Chicago: Year Book, 1989:255-259.

99. Dickersin, K, et al. Publication bias and clinical trials. Controlled Clin Trials 1987;8:343-353.

100. Dickersin, K and Min, Y-I. Publication bias: the problem that won't go away. In: Doing more good than harm: the evaluation of health care inteventions: NY: Annals of the NYAS, 1993:135-148.

101. Dietz, D. Science and the American press (12/29/36). Quoted in: Lewis, HJ. Science and media then and now...a world apart. ScienceWriters 1995;42:1-4.

102. DiMaggio, JR, et al. Hallucinations and ifosfamide-induced neurotoxicity. Cancer 1994;73:1509-1514.

103. DiMario, FJJ and Packer, RJ. Acute mental status changes in children with systemic cancer. Pediatrics 1990;85:353-360.

104. Dollinger, M, et al. [eds.] Everyone's guide to cancer therapy. Kansas City: Andrews & McMeel, 1991.

105. Dreizen, S, et al. Nutritional deficiencies in patients receiving cancer chemotherapy. Postgrad Med. 1990;87:163-167, 170.

106. Drings, P, et al. [Chemotherapy of the non-small cell carcinoma of the lung with ifosfamide and cisplatin.] Dtsch Med Wochenschr 1984;109:1059-1064.

107. Durrant, KR, et al. Comparison of treatment policies in inoperable bronchial carcinoma. Lancet 1971;1:715-719.

108. Early Breast Cancer Trialists' Collaborative Group. Systemic treatment of early breast cancer by hormonal, cytotoxic, or immune therapy. Lancet 1992;339:1-15, 71-85.

109. Ebeling, K and Spitzbart, H. [Registration of cytostatic effects on cultured cells in vitro and their current significance for individualized chemotherapy of tumors in advanced ovarian carcinoma.] Zentralbl Gynakol 1977;99:1041-1054.

110. Edmondson, JH, et al. Cyclophosphamide and CCNU in the treatment of inoperable small cell lung cancer and adenocarcinoma of the lung. Cancer Treat Rep 1973;60:925-932.

111. Ehrlich, P. The collected papers of Paul Ehrlich. F. Himmelweit, ed. London: Pergamon, 1956.

112. Einhorn, LH, et al. Cancer of the testis. In: DeVita, 1993:1126-1151.

113. Einzig, AI, et al. Phase II trial of taxol in patients with metastatic renal cell carcinoma. Cancer Invest 1991;9:133-136.

114. Endicott, K. Interview, National Library of Medicine, 1964. In: Patterson, 1987:196.

115. Epstein, SS and Rennie, SA. Travesty at women's expense. Los Angeles Times. 6/22/92.

REFERENCES

116. Ettinger, DS, et al. Phase II study of PALA and PCNU in the treatment of non-small cell lung cancer (NSCLC). Cancer Treat Rep 1984;68:1297-1298.

117. Evans, KT. Breast cancer symposium: points in the practical management of breast cancer. Are physical methods of diagnosis of value? Brit J Surg 1969; 56:784-786.

118. Feinleib, M and Zelen, M. Some pitfalls in the evaluation of screening programs. Arch Environ Health 1969;19:412-415.

119. Feinstein, AR, et al. The Will Rogers phenomenon: stage migration and new diagnostic techniques as a source of misleading statistics for survival in cancer. NEJM 1985;312:1604-1608.

120. Fields, KK, et al. Maximum-tolerated doses of ifosfamide, carboplatin, and etoposide given over 6 days followed by autologous stem-cell rescue: toxicity profile. JCO 1995;13:323-332.

121. Finkelstein, JZ. Childhood cancers. In: Dollinger, 1991.

122. Fisher, B, et al. Surgical adjuvant chemotherapy in cancer of the breast. Ann Surg 1968;168:337-356.

123. Fisher, B, et al. A randomized clinical trial evaluating sequential methotrexate and fluorouracil in the treatment of patients with node negative breast cancer who have estrogen receptor negative tumors. NEJM 1989;320:473-478.

124. Fisher, B, et al. A randomized clinical trial evaluating tamoxifen in the treatment of patients with node negative breast cancer who have estrogen receptor positive tumors. NEJM 320:479-484.

125. Forkner, CE. Leukemia and allied disorders. NY: Macmillan, 1938.

126. Fornander, T., et al. Effects of tamoxifen on the female genital tract. Ann NY Acad Sci 1991;622:469-476.

127. Foti, M. 'Research cures cancer' national public education campaign to premier in Washington, DC on January 25, 1995 [media release]. Washington, DC: The National Coalition for Cancer Research, 1/24/95.

128. Franks, LM. Latency and progression in tumors: the natural history of prostatic cancer. Lancet 1956;ii:1037-1039.

129. Frey, C, et al. Randomized study of 5-FU and CCNU in pancreatic cancer. Cancer 1981;47:27-31.

130. Fritze, D, et al. A randomized study of combination chemotherapy (VAC-FMC) with or without immunstimulation by corynebacterium parvum in metastastic breast cancer. Klin Wochenschr 1982;60:593-598.

131. Frost & Sullivan. World cancer therapeutics markets [executive summary]. Mountain View, CA: Frost & Sullivan, 1993.

132. Fuks, JZ, et al. Randomized study of cyclophosphamide, doxorubicin and etoposide with or without cisplatinum in non-small cell lung cancer. JCO. 1983;1:295-301.

133. Garewal, HS. Beta-carotene and vitamin E in oral cancer prevention. J Cell Biochem Suppl 1993;17S:262-269.

134. Garewal, HS. Potential role of beta-carotene and antioxidant vitamins in the prevention of oral cancer. Ann N Y Acad Sci 1992:260-268.

135. Gehan, EA and Lemark, NA. Statistics in medical research: developments in clinical trials. NY: Plenum,1994.

136. Ghussen F, et al. The role of regional hyperthermic cytostatic perfusion in the treatment of extremity melanoma. Cancer 1988;61:654-659.

137. Ghussen, F, et al. Hyperthermic perfusion with chemotherapy for melanoma of the extremities. World Journal of Surgery 1989;13:598-602.

138. Gill, PS, et al. Systemic treatment of AIDS-related Kaposi's sarcoma: results of a randomized trial. Amer J Med 1991;90:427-433.

139. Gill, TM and Feinstein, AR. A critical appraisal of the quality of quality-of-life measurements [see comments]. JAMA 1994;272:619-626.

140. Gilman, A. The initial clinical trial of nitrogen mustard. Am J Surg 1963;105: 574-578.

141. Ginsberg, RJ, et al. Cancer of the lung. In: DeVita, 1993:673-758.

142. Glass, A, et al. Acute toxicity during adjuvant chemotherapy for breast cancer: The NSABP experience from 1717 patients receiving single and multiple agents. Cancer Treat Rep 1981;65:363-376.

143. Glassberg, AB. Lung: non-small cell. In: Dollinger, 1991:404-410.

144. Glassman, J. The cancer survivors and how they did it. NY: The Dial Press, 1983.

145. Glemser, B. Man against cancer. NY: Funk and Wagnalls, 1969.

146. Goffman, E. The presentation of self in everyday life. NY: Doubleday, 1959.

147. Goldie, JH. Scientific basis for adjuvant and primary (neoadjuvant) chemotherapy. Seminars in Oncol 1987;14:1-7.

148. Golomb, FM. Agents used in cancer chemotherapy. Am J Surg 1963;105:579-590.

149. Goodman, PM, et al. Cost-effectiveness of cancer chemotherapy: an economic evaluation of a randomized trial in small-cell lung cancer. JCO 1988;6:1537-1547.

150. Govallo, VI. Immunology of pregnancy and cancer. Commack, NY: Nova, 1993.

151. Grace, ND, et al. The present status of portal hypertension in cirrhosis. Gastroenterology 1966;50:684-691.

152. Gray, D, et al. A comparative cost analysis of terminal cancer care in home hospice patients and controls. J Chronic Dis 1987;40:801-810.

153. Greco, RA, et al. Rationale for chemotherapy for patients with advanced non-small-cell lung cancer. Sem in Oncol 1986;13(Suppl. 3):92-96.

154. Green, RA, et al. Alkylating agents in bronchogenic carcinoma. Am J Med 1969; 46:516-525.

155. Greenberg, D. A critical look at cancer coverage. CJR 1975; Jan-Feb:40-44.

156. Greenberg, D. Progress in cancer research—don't say it isn't so. NEJM 1975;292: 707-708.

157. Greene, D, et al. A comparison of patient-reported side effects among three chemotherapy regimens for breast cancer. Cancer Practice 1994;2:57-62.

158. Greene, M, et al. Acute nonlymphocytic leukemia after therapy with alkylating agents for ovarian cancer. NEJM 1982;307:1416-1421.

159. Gribel, NV and Pashinskii, VG. [Antimetastatic properties of aloe juice.] Vopr Onkol 1986;32:38-40.

160. Gutin, PH. Is chemotherapy useful in the most frequently encountered brain tumors? In: Wiernik, PH. [ed.] Controv. in Oncology. NY: Wiley, 1982:207-219.

161. Haines, IE, et al. Very high dose cisplatin (CDDP) with bleomycin (BLEO) by 24-hour continuous infusion (CI) in advanced squamous cancer of the head and neck; no dose-response relationship. Proc Amer Assoc Cancer Res 1987;28:217.

162. Hall, MB. Robert Boyle on natural philosophy. Bloomington: IUP,1965:121.

163. Hanks, GE, et al. Cancer of the prostate. In: DeVita, 1993:1073-1113.

164. Hansen, HH, et al. Combination chemotherapy of advanced lung cancer. Cancer 1976;38:2201-2207.

165. Hansen, HH, et al. Chemotherapy of advanced small cell anaplastic carcinoma: superiority of a four-drug combination to a three-drug combination. Ann Intern Med 1978;89:177-181.

166. Hansen, HH. Advanced non-small cell lung cancer: to treat or not to treat? JCO 1987;5:1711-1712.

167. Hardy, R and Horning, S. Lymphoma: Hodgkin's disease. In: Dollinger, 1991.

168. Hartunian, NS, et al. The incidence and economic costs of cancer, motor vehicle injuries, coronary heart disease, and stroke: a comparative analysis. Am J Public Health 1980;70:1249-1260.

169. Haskell, CM. Pros and cons of chemotherapy. Los Angeles Times. 1/22/87.

170. Haskell, CM. Chemotherapy and survival of patients with non-small cell lung cancer: a contrary view. Chest 1991;99:1325-1326.

171. He, J, et al. [Effects of mixture of astragalus membranaceus, fructus ligustri lucidi and eclipta prostrata on immune function in mice.] Hua Hsi I Ko Ta Hsueh Hsueh Pao 1992;23:408-411.

172. Henderson, IC and Canellos, GP. Cancer of the breast: the past decade. NEJM 1980;302:17-30, 78-90.

173. Henderson, IC, et al. New agents and new medical treatments for advanced breast cancer. Semin Oncol 1987;14:34-64.

174. Henderson, IC. Stehen ansprechraten und dauer des uberlebens in kausaler beziehung? In: Onkologisches kolloquium therapiestrategien beim metas-tasierenden mammakarzinom. Berlin: Walter de Gruyer, 1987.

175. Herrmann, R, et al. Sequential methotrexate and 5-fluorouracil: improved response rate in metastatic colorectal cancer. JCO 1984;2:591-594.

176. Hildebrand, J and Delecluse, F. Malignant glioma. In: Slevin and Staquet, 1986:583-604.

177. Hill, DL. A review of cyclophosphamide. Springfield, IL: Thomas, 1975.

178. Hillemanns, HG. Das fortgeschrittene genitalkarzinom. Das inkurable karzinom. das karzinomrezidiv. Munich: Urban & Schwarzenberg, 1981.

179. Hilts, PJ. US Breast cancer deaths fell nearly 5 percent in three years. New York Times. 1/13/95.

180. Hockey, MS and Fielding, JWL. Gastric cancer. In: Slevin and Staquet, 1986.

181. Hodgson, TA and Rice, DP. Economic impact of cancer in the United States. In: Schottenfeld, D and Fraumeni, JF [eds.] Cancer epidemiology and prevention. Philadelphia: Saunders, 1982:208-228.

182. Hoffmann, PC, et al. Chemotherapy of metastatic non-small cell bronchogenic carcinoma. Semin Oncol 1983;10:111-122.

183. Holmes, FA, et al. Phase II Trial of taxol: an active drug in metastatic breast cancer. JNCI 1991;83:1797-1805.

184. Horsman, MR, et al. Changes in the response of the RIF-1 tumour to melphalan in vivo induced by inhibitors of nuclear ADP-ribosyl transferase. Br J Cancer 1986;53:247-254.

185. Houston, BL. Pros and cons on chemotherapy. LA Times. 1/22/87.

186. Houston, SJ, et al. The influence of adjuvant chemotherapy on outcome after relapse in patients with breast cancer. Proc Annu Meet ASCO 1992;11:A108.

187. Hreschchyshyn, MM, et al. Hydroxyurea or placebo combined with radiation to treat stages IIIb and IV in cervical cancer confined to the pelvis. J Radiat Oncol Biol Phys 1979;5:317-322.

188. Hrushesky, WJM and Bjarnason, GA. The application of circadian chronobiology to cancer chemotherapy. In: DeVita, 1993:2666-2686.

189. Hurteloup, P, et al. Phase II trial of idarubicin in advanced breast cancer. Eur J Ca Clin Oncol 1989;25:423-428.

190. Hutchison, GB and Shapiro, S. Lead time gained by diagnostic screening for breast cancer. JNCI 1968;41:666-673.

191. Illich, I. Medical nemesis: the expropriation of health. NY: Bantam Books, 1976.

192. Information Please Almanac (electronic version). Cancer in the 21st century. Boston: Houghton Mifflin, 1994.

193. Israel, L. Conquering cancer. NY: Random House, 1978.

194. James, JD, et al. A guide to drug interactions. NY: McGraw Hill, 1978.

195. Jarabak, J and Rice, K. Metastatic adrenal cortical carcinoma, prolonged regression with mitotane therapy. JAMA 1981;246:1706.

196. Jebb, SA, et al. 5-fluorouracil and folinic acid-induced mucositis: no effect of oral glutamine supplementation. Br J Cancer 1994;70:732-735.

197. Johnson, JR and Templer, R. FDA requirements for approval of new anti-cancer drugs. Cancer Treat Rep 1985;69:1155-1157.

198. Jonat, W, et al. Chemo- or endocrine adjuvant therapy alone or combined in post-menopausal patients (GABG Trial 1). Rec Results Cancer Res 1989;115:163-169.

199. Jones, AL and Miller, JL. Bone marrow morbidity of chemotherapy. In: Complications of Cancer Management Oxford: Butterworth, 1991;379-397.

200. Jönsson, B and Karlsson, G. Economic evaluation of cancer treatments. In: Williams, CJ [ed.] Introducing new treatments for cancer: practical, ethical and legal problems. NY: John Wiley & Sons, 1992.

201. Joslyn, AF. Ondansetron, clinical development for postoperative nausea and vomiting: current studies and future directions. Anaesthesia 1994;49S:34-37.

202. Kagan, BM, et al. Spotlight on antimicrobial agents. JAMA 1973;226:306-310.

203. Kamen, BA, et al. Ifosamide: should the honeymoon be over? JCO 1995;13:307-309.

204. Karnofsky, D. Cancer chemotherapeutic agents. CA Cancer J Clin 1968;18:72-79.

205. Karnofsky, D. New drugs for the treatment of cancer. In: Ross, W. The climate is hope: Englewood Cliffs, NJ: Prentice-Hall, 1965:126.

206. Kaufman, RJ. Advanced breast cancer. Cancer 1981;47:2398-2403.

207. Kaufmann, M, et al. Adjuvant chemo- and endocrine therapy alone or in combination in premenopausal patients. Rec Results Cancer Res 1989;115:118-125.

208. Kaufmann, M, et al. Adjuvant randomized trials of doxorubicin/cyclophosphamide vs. doxorubicin/cyclophosphamide/tamoxifen and CMF chemotherapy vs. tamoxifen in women with node-positive breast cancer. JCO 1993;11:454-460.

209. Kennedy, MJ, et al. High-dose chemotherapy with reinfusion of purged autologous bone marrow following dose-intense induction... JNCI 1991;83:920-926.

210. Kidd, JG. Regression of transplanted lymphomas in vivo by means of normal guinea pig serum. J Exp Med 1953;98:565-582.

211. Kolata, G. Women resist trials to test marrow transplants. New York Times, 2/15/95.

212. Koren, G. Bias against negative studies in newspaper reports of medical research. JAMA 1991;266:1824-1826.

213. Koyama, M, et al. Novel type of potential anti-cancer agents derived from chrysophanol and emodin. Some structure-activity relationship studies. J Med Chem 1988;31:283-284.

214. Koyama, M, et al. Intercalating agents with covalent bond forming capability. A novel type of potential anti-cancer agent. Derivatives of chrysophanol and emodin. J Med Chem 1989;32:1594-1599.

215. Kris, M, et al. Delayed emesis following anti-cancer chemotherapy. Support Care Cancer 1994;2:297-300.

216. Kristof, NB. When doctors won't tell cancer patients the truth. NY Times, 2/25/95.

217. Krokon, O, et al. Ifosfamide vs. ifosfamide and CCNU in the treatment of inoperable small cell lung cancer. Onkologie 1982;5:56-59.

218. Krumbharr, EB. Role of the blood and the bone marrow in certain forms of gas poisoning. I. Peripheral blood changes and their significance. JAMA 1919;131:39.

219. Kushner, R. Is aggressive adjuvant chemotherapy the Halsted of the '80s? CA Cancer Jour Clin 1984;34:345-351.

220. Lad, TE, et al. Immediate vs. postponed chemotherapy (CAMP) for unresectable non small cell lung cancer: a randomized trial. Cancer Treatment Reports 1981; 65:973-978.

221. Laing, AH, et al. Treatment of inoperable carcinoma of bronchus. Lancet 1971;2:1161-1165.

222. Laing, AH, et al. Treatment of small-cell carcinomas of the bronchus. Lancet 1975;1:129-132.

223. Lambe, M, et al. Transient increase in the risk of breast cancer after giving birth. NEJM 1994;331:5-9.

224. Landers, A. Few find chemotherapy to be a day at the beach. Chi. Trib., 12/10/90.

225. Laszlo, J. Understanding cancer. NY: Harper & Row, 1987.

226. Lavin, P, et al. Survival and response to chemotherapy for advanced colorectal adenocarcinoma. Cancer 1980;46:1536-1543.

227. Lejeune, FJ. Malignant melanoma. In: Slevin and Staquet, 1986: 549-559.

228. Lerner, I., et al. The prevalence of questionable methods of cancer treatment in the United States. CA Cancer Jour Clin 1992;42:181-191.

229. Levin, L and Hryniuk, WM. Dose intensity analysis of chemotherapy regimens in ovarian cancer. JCO 1987;5:756-767.

230. Levin, VA, et al. Neoplasms of the central nervous system. In: DeVita, 1993: 1679-1737.

231. Lippman, SM, et al. Retinoids in chemoprevention of head and neck carcinogenesis. Prev Med 1993;22:693-700.

232. Loeb, S. Chemotherapy handbook. Springhouse, PA: Springhouse Corp., 1994.

233. Loprinzi, CI and Ahmann, DL. Chemotherapy vs. hormonal therapy in advanced breast carcinoma [correspondence]. NEJM 1986;315:1092-1093.

234. Lowenbraun, S, et al. Combination chemotherapy in small cell lung carcinoma: a randomized study of two intensive regimes. Cancer 1984;54:2344-2350.

235. Lucas, KG, et al. Cardiorespiratory decompensation following methylprednisolone administration. Pediatr Hematol Oncol 1993;10:249-255.

236. Ludlum, DB. Therapeutic agents as potential carcinogens. 1990; In: Grover, PL and Cooper, CS [eds.] Chemical carcinogenesis and mutagenesis I. Berlin: Springer-Verlag, 1990:153-175.

237. Ludwig Breast Cancer Study Group. Toxic effects of early adjuvant chemotherapy for breast cancer. Lancet 1983;2:542-544.

238. Ludwig Breast Cancer Study Group. Prolonged disease-free interval after one course of perioperative adjunctive chemotherapy for node negative breast cancer. NEJM 1989;320:491-496.

239. Lundberg, GD. Communicating science and health in the new millenium. In: Lewis, HJ. Science and media then and now. ScienceWriters 1994-1995;42:14.

240. Lung Cancer Study Group, The. The benefit of adjuvant treatment for resected locally advanced non-small-cell lung cancer. JCO 1988;6:9-17.

241. Macaulay, V and Smith, IE. Advanced breast cancer. In: Slevin and Staquet, 1986: 273-258.

242. MacBurney, M, et al. A cost-evaluation of glutamine-supplemented parenteral nutrition in adult bone marrow transplant patients. J Am Diet Assoc 1994;94:1263-1266.

243. Mackillop, WJ, et al. The use of expert surrogates to evaluate clinical trials in non-small cell lung cancer. Br J Cancer 1986;54:661-667.

244. Maguire, GP, et al. Psychiatric morbidity and physical toxicity associated with adjuvant chemotherapy after mastectomy. Br J Med 1980;281:1179-1180.

245. Malik, STA. Small cell lung cancer. In: Slevin and Staquet, 1986: 493-524.

246. Mallison, CN, et al. Chemotherapy in pancreatic cancer: results of a controlled, prospective, randomized, multicentre trial. Brit Med J 1980;281:1589-1591.

247. Mansour, EG, et al. Efficacy of adjuvant chemotherapy in high risk node negative breast cancer: an intergroup study. NEJM 1989;320:485-490.

248. Marselos, M and Vainio, H. Carcinogenic properties of pharmaceutical agents evaluated in the IARC monographs programme. Carcinogenesis 1991;12:1751-1766.

249. Marshall, E. Broder to join exodus from NCI. Science 1995;267:24.

250. Marshall, E. Fisher clashes with NCI—again. Science 1995;267:954.

251. McCardle, CS, et al. The social, emotional and financial implications of adjuvant chemotherapy in breast cancer. Br J Surg 1981;68:261-264.

252 McGuire, WL. Adjuvant therapy for node-negative breast cancer. NEJM 1989; 320:525-527.

253. McGuire, WP, et al. Taxol: a unique antineoplastic agent with significant activity in advanced ovarian epithelial neoplasms. Ann Intern Med 1989;111:273-279.

254. McKinnon, NE. The effects of control programs on cancer mortality. Can Med Assoc J 1960;82:1308-1312.

255. McMillan, TJ and Hart, IR. Can cancer chemotherapy enhance the malignant behavior of tumors? Cancer and Metas Rev 1987;6:503-520.

256. McNeil Pharmaceuticals. Entry on "haldol" In: Physicians desk reference, 46th Ed., Montvale, NJ: Medical Economics Co., 1992:1376.

257. McNeil, BJ, et al. Speech and survival tradeoffs between quality and quantity of life in laryngeal cancer. NEJM 1981;305:982-987.

258. Mehta, C and Vogl, SE. High-dose cyclophosphamide in the induction chemotherapy of small cell lung cancer. Minor improvements in rate of remission and survival. Proc Am Assoc for Ca Res 1982;23:155.

259. Meisenberg BR, et al. Randomized trial of high-dose chemotherapy with autologous bone marrow support as adjuvant therapy for high-risk, multi-node-positive malignant melanoma. JNCI 1993;85:1080-1085.

260. Miller, BA, et al. [eds.] SEER cancer statistics review: 1973-1990 (NIH Pub. No. 93-2789), Bethesda, MD: NCI, 1993.

261. Miller, RW and McKay, FW. Decline in the US childhood cancer mortality: 1950 to 1980. JAMA 1984;251:1567-1570.

262. Miyaji, NT. The power of compassion: truth-telling among American doctors in the care of dying patients. Soc Sci Med 1993;36:249-264.

263. Miyaji, NT. Informed consent, cancer, and truth in prognosis [letter]. NEJM 1994;331:810.

264. Moertel, CG, et al. Combined 5-fluorouracil and supervoltage radiation therapy of locally unresectable gastrointestinal cancer. Lancet 1969;ii:865-867.

265. Moertel, CG, et al. Levamisole and fluorouracil for adjuvant therapy of resected colon carcinoma. NEJM 1990;322:352-358.

266. Moertel, CG, et al. The intergroup study of fluorouracil (5-FU) plus levamisole (LEV) and levamisole alone as adjuvant therapy for stage C colon cancer: a final report. Proc ASCO 1992;11:161.

267. Moore, G, et al. Chemotherapy as an adjuvant to surgery. Amer J Surg 1963;105:591-597.

268. Moore, MJ and Tannock, IJ. How expert physicians would wish to be treated if they developed genito-urinary cancer (Abstract No. 455). Proc ASCO 1988;7:118.

269. Moss, RW. The cancer industry, NY: Paragon, 1989. (Distrib. by Equinox Press)

270. Moss, RW. Big money in new cancer drugs. The Cancer Chronicles 1991;2:4-5.

271. Moss, RW. Cancer therapy: the independent consumer's guide to non-toxic treatment and prevention. Brooklyn, NY: Equinox Press, 1994.

272. Mutch, RS and Hutson, PR. Levamisole in the adjuvant treatment of colon cancer [review]. Clinical Pharmacy 1991;10:95-109.

273. Myers, C, et al. Suramin: a novel growth factor antagonist with activity in hormone-refractory metastatic prostate cancer. JCO 1990;8:1830-1838.

274. Myers, MH. Breast cancer survival over three decades. In: Griem, ML [ed.] Breast cancer: a challenging problem. NY: Springer, 1973:87-91.

275. National Cancer Institute, PDQ. Statement on colon cancer, 4/14/94.

276. National Cancer Institute, PDQ. Reanalyses of NSABP protocols B06, B13, B14, 6/5/94.

277. National Cancer Institute, PDQ. Statement on malignant melanoma, 2/2/95.

278. National Cancer Institute, PDQ. Breast cancer statement, 2/15/95.

279. National Institutes of Health. NIH consensus-development statement: adjuvant chemotherapy of breast cancer. NEJM 1980;303:831-832.

280. National Institutes of Health. NIH consensus conference: treatment of early stage breast cancer. JAMA 1991;265:391-395.

281. Nealon, TFJ. Low-grade tumors of the breast do not require adjuvant therapy. ACS's 32nd Science Writers Seminar, 3/27/90.

282. Neergaard, L. FDA—cancer drug. Associated Press, 12/16/94.

283. Neijt, JP, et al. Randomized trial comparing two combination chemotherapy regimens in advanced ovarian cancer. Lancet 1984;ii:594-600.

284. Neijt, JP, et al. Long-term results of combination chemotherapy in advanced ovarian cancer (Abstract No. 526). Proc ASCO 1988;7:136.

285. Norton, JA, et al. Cancer of the endocrine system. In: DeVita,1993:1333-1435.

286. Nuter, LM, et al. Menadione: spectrum of anticancer activity and effects on nucleotide metabolism in human antineoplastic cell lines. Biochem Pharmacol 1991;41:1283-1292.

287. O'Regan, B and Hirschberg, C. Spontaneous remission: an annotated bibliography. Sausalito: Institute of Noetic Sciences, 1993.

288. Oeser, H. Krebsbekämpfung: hoffnung und realität. Stuttgart: Thieme, 1974.

289. Olivotto, IA, et al. Adjuvant systemic therapy and survival after breast cancer NEJM. 1994;330:805-810.

290. Osterlind, K, et al. Treatment of advanced small cell carcinoma of the lung: continuous vs. alternating combination chemotherapy. Can Res 1985;43:6085-6089.

291. Oye RK and Shapiro MF. Reporting from chemotherapy trials. Does response make a difference in patient survival? JAMA 1984;252:2722-2725.

292. Pack, GT and Livingston, EM. Treatment of cancer and allied diseases, by 147 international authors. NY: Paul B. Hoeber, 1940.

293. Palmer, MK. Survival studies using a computer-based hospital registry of 29,000 cancer patients. In: Tagnon, HJ and Staquet, MJ [eds.]; Controversies in Cancer: Design of Trials and Treatment. New York: Masson Publishing USA, 1979.

294. Pannuti, F, et al. High dose cyclophosphamide vs. cyclophosphamide, methotrexate, 5FU and hydroxyurea (CMFH) in the treatment of stage III non-small cell bronchogenic carcinoma: a randomized trial. Cancer Treat Rep 1980; 64:1131-1134.

295. Patterson, JT. The dread disease. Cambridge, MA: Harvard University Press, 1987.

296. Pauling, L. How to live longer and feel better. NY: WH Freeman & Co., 1986.

297. Paulos, JA. Counting on dyscalculia. Discover 3/94:30-36.

298. Perry, MC and Yarbro, JW. Toxicity of chemotherapy. Orlando: Grune & Stratton, 1984.

299. Petru, E and Schmahl, D. No relevant influence on overall survival time in patients with metastatic breast cancer undergoing combination chemotherapy. J Cancer Res Clin Oncol 1988;114:183-185.

300. Piccirillo, JF, et al. New clinical severity staging system for cancer of the larynx. Five-year survival rates. Ann Otol Rhinol Laryngol 1994;103:83-92.

301. Piver, MS, et al. Hydroxyurea: a radiation potentiator in carcinoma of the uterine cervix. Amer J Obstet Gynecol 1983;147:803-808.

302. Pizzo, PA, et al. Cancers in children. In: Wittes, 1991.

303. Pizzo, PA, et al. Solid tumors of childhood. In: DeVita, 1993:1738-1791.

304. Plowman, PN, et al. Introduction. In: Plowman, PN, et al. [eds.], Complicatons of cancer management. Oxford: Butterworth-Heinemann, 1991.

305. Pocock, SJ. Clinical trials: a practical approach. NY: Wiley & Sons, 1984.

306. Pollner, F. Data support adjuvant therapy. Medical World News 1989;80-85.

307. Possinger, K, et al. Chemotherapie metastasierter mammakarzinome. Dt Med Wschr 1988;113:224-230.

308. Pourquier, H. The results of adjuvant chemotherapy are predominantly caused by the hormonal changes such therapy induces. in: Van Scoy-Mosher, 1981: 83-99.

309. Powles, TJ, et al. Failure of chemotherapy to prolong survival in a group of patients with metastatic breast cancer. Lancet 1980;i:580-582.

310. Powles, TJ. In: von Fournier, D and Kubli, F. [eds.], Growth behavior and implications for staging and therapy. Berlin: Springer-Verlag, 1989.

311. Quirt, IC, et al. Improved survival in patients with poor-prognosis malignant melanoma treated with adjuvant levamisole: a phase III study by the National Cancer Institute of Canada Clinical Trials Group. JCO 1991;9:729-735.

312. Radner, G. It's always something. NY: Simon and Schuster, 1989.

313. Raghavan, D. Chemotherapy for advanced bladder cancer: 'Midsummer Night's Dream' or 'Much Ado About Nothing'? Br J Cancer 1990;62:337-340.

314. Rankin, EM. Non-small-cell lung cancer. In: Slevin and Staquet, 1986: 447-491.

315. Redmond, C., et al. The methodological dilemma in retrospectively correlating the amount of chemotherapy received in adjuvant therapy protocols with disease-free survival. Cancer Treat Rep 1983;67:519-526.

316. Reed, E. Platinum analogs. In: DeVita, 1993:390-417.

317. Rees, GJ. Cost-effectiveness in oncology. Lancet 1985;ii:1405-1407.

318. Rhoads, CP, et al. Triethylene melamine in the treatment of Hodgkin's disease and allied neoplasms. Tr A Am Physicians 1950;63:136.

319. Rhoads, CP. Dependence of medicine on industrial invention and research. Memorial Hospital press release, 3/8/40.

320. Richards, et al. Adjuvant chemotherapy with doxorubicin and 5-fluorouracil in T3, Nx, M0 bladder cancer treated with radiotherapy. Br J Urol 1983;55:386-391.

321. Richards, V. Cancer: the wayward cell. Berkeley: U of Calif Press,1972:215.

322. Ries, LAG, et al. Cancer statistics review 1973-1990, Bethesda: NCI,1990.

323. Ries, LAG, et al. SEER cancer statistics review, 1973-1991: Tables and Graphs. Bethesda: NCI, 1994.

324. Rimer, I. The mass media and the cancer patient—some views. Health Education Quarterly 1984;10:95-100.

325. Rinsky, RA, et al. Benzene and leukemia. NEJM 1987;316:1044.

326. Roberts, JT and Hall, RR. The role of chemotherapy in the treatment of bladder cancer. In: Tumours in urology, London: Springer, 1994.

327. Rosenbaum, EH and Dollinger, M. Stomach. In: Dollinger, 1991:515-524.

328. Rosenbaum, EH. Anus. In: Dollinger, 1991:210-215.

329. Rowinsky, EK, et al. Phase I and pharmacodynamic study of taxol in refractory acute leukemias. JCO 1991;9:1704-1712.

330. Rubens, RD, et al. Controlled trial of adjuvant chemotherapy with melphalan for breast cancer. Lancet 1983;i:839-843.

331. Russo, RV. New York Times [letter], 4/5/94.

332. Sarna, GP. Pros and cons of chemotherapy. Los Angeles Times, 2/22/87.

333. Scarfe, MA and Israel, MK. Possible drug interaction between warfarin and combination of levamisole and fluorouracil. Ann Pharmacother 1994;28:464-467.

334. Schadendorf, D, et al. Chemosensitivity testing of human malignant melanoma: a retrospective analysis of clinical response and in vitro drug sensitivity. Cancer 1994;73:103-108.

335. Schipper, H. Treating cancer: is kill cure? Ann Acad Med Singapore 1994;23:382-386.

336. Schipper, H and Dick, JAD. Does consensus help in breast cancer? Lancet 1994;344:836.

337. Schneider, SM and Distelhorst, CW. Chemotherapy-induced emergencies. Seminars in Oncology 1989;16:572-578.

338. Schnitzler, G, et al. Prospektiv randomisierte prufung von 5-fluorouracil, adriamycin, BCNU (FAB) vs. beobachtung beim metastasierten prancreaskarzinom. Tumor Diagnostik und Therapie 1986;7:135-138.

339. Selaway, O, et al. Methotrexate compared with placebo in lung cancer. Cancer 1977;40:4-8.

340. Shapiro, M. Chemotherapy: snake-oil remedy? It has its purposes but use is dubious in some cancers. Los Angeles Times, 1/9/87.

341. Shearer, RJ, et al. Adjuvant chemotherapy in carcinoma of the bladder. A prospective trial preliminary report. Br J Urol 1988;62:558-564.

342. Shimkin, MB. Contrary to nature (DHEW Publication No. NIH 79-720). Bethesda: NCI, 1979.

343. Simes, RJ. Publication bias: the case for an international registry of clinical trials. JCO 1986;4:1529-1541.

344. Simone, CB. Cancer and nutrition. Garden City Park: Avery, 1994.

345. Simone, CB. "Conventional" systemic treatments. Chapter 22 of a forthcoming book on breast cancer. (Garden City Park: Avery). (Our thanks to Dr. Simone for allowing us to preview this book in manuscript.)

346. Slevin, ML and Staquet, MJ. Randomized trials in cancer: a critical review by sites. Monograph series of the European Organization for Research (EORTC) on Treatment of Cancer. NY: Raven Press, 1986.

347. Slevin, ML. Ovarian cancer. In: Slevin and Staquet, 1986.

348. Smigel, K. Experts agree to disagree on adjuvant therapy for breast cancer. JNCI 1990;82:640-641.

349. Solar, S, et al. [Immunostimulating properties of an extract isolated and partially purified from aloe vahombe.] Arch Inst Pasteur Madagascar 1980;47:9-39.

350. Soquet, Y. Combined surgery and adjuvant chemotherapy with high dose methotrexate and folinic acid rescue (HDMTX-CF) for infiltrating tumours of the bladder. Br J Urol 1981;53:439-443.

351. Sorensen, JB and Hansen, HH. Is there a role for vindesine in the treatment of non-small cell lung cancer? Invest New Drugs 1993;11:103-133.

352. Spitler, LE. A randomized trial of levamisole versus placebo as adjuvant therapy in malignant melanoma. JCO 1991;9:736-740.

353. Stahl, M, et al. Lonidamine vs. high-dose tamoxifen in progressive, advanced renal cell carcinoma: results of an ongoing randomized phase II study. Semin Oncol 1991;18(2 suppl 4):33-37.

354. Standard S and Nathan, H. Should the patient know the truth? NY: Springer Publishing Co., 1955.

355. Steele, GDJ, et al. National cancer data base: annual review of patient care. Atlanta: American Cancer Society, 1994.

356. Stern, J L. Ovary. In: Dollinger, 1991.

357. Stokes, J. Certain technical requirements in methods of intravenous injections. Med Rec 1917;92:529.

358. Szczepanska, I, et al. Inhibition of leukocyte migration by cancer chemotherapeutic agents and its prevention by free radical scavengers and thiols. Eur J Hematol 1988;40:69-74.

359. Tannock, IF. A randomized trial of two dose levels of cyclophosphamide, methotrexate, and fluorouracil chemotherapy for patients with metastatic breast cancer. JCO 1988;6:1377-1387.

360. Tattersall, MHN and Friedlander, ML. Cost considerations in cancer chemotherapy. Aust Health Rev 1982;5:21-24.

361. Taylor I, et al. A randomized controlled trial of adjuvant portal vein cytotoxic perfusion in colorectal cancer. Brit J Surg 1985;72:359-363.

362. Taylor, SG, et al. Combination chemotherapy vs. tamoxifen as initial therapy forstage IV breast cancer in elderly women. Ann Int Med. 1986;104:455-461.

363. ten Bokkel, HWW. Current status of chemotherapy for ovarian cancer. Eur J Cancer Clin Oncol. 1988;24:583-585.

364. Thigpen, JT, et al. Chemotherapy for advanced or recurrent gynecological cancer. Cancer 1987;60:2104-2116.

365. Thorp-Stanley, R. Pros and cons on chemotherapy. Los Angeles Times, 1/22/87.

366. Todd, M, et al. Survival of women with metastatic breast cancer at Yale from 1920 to 1980. JCO 1983;1:406-408.

367. Tonato, M, et al. Antiemetics in cancer chemotherapy: historical perspective and current state of the art. Support Care Cancer 1994;2:150-160.

368. Tonato, M, et al. Are there differences among the serotonin antagonists? Support Care Cancer 1994;2:293-296.

369. Tonkin, K and Tannock, I. Evaluation of response and morbidity following treatment of bladder cancer. In: Raghaven, D [ed.] The Management of Bladder Cancer, Baltimore: Williams & Wilkins, 1988:228-244.

370. Torti, FM and Lum, BL. The biology and treatment of superficial bladder cancer. JCO 1984;2:505-531.

371. Trugman, J, et al. Cisplatin neurotoxicity: failure to demonstrate Vitamin B12 inactivation. Cancer Treat Rep 1985;69:453-455.

372. UICC (International Union Against Cancer). Manual of clinical oncology. Berlin: Springer-Verlag, 1982.

373. US Congress, Office of Technology Assessment. The impact of randomized clinical trials on health policy and medical practice. Washington, DC, 1983.

374. US Department of Commerce. 1992 Census of manufactures, preliminary report, industry series. Washington, DC, 1992.

375. US Department of Health and Human Services. HHS news: breast cancer deaths decline nearly 5 percent. Washington, DC, 1995.

376. Van Scoy-Mosher, MB [ed.] Medical oncology: controversies in cancer treatment. Boston: GK Hall, 1981.

377. van Slooten, H, et al. The treatment of adenocortical carcinoma with o,p-DDD: prognostic implications of serum levels monitoring. Eur J Cancer Clin Oncol 1984;20:47-53.

378. van Zaanen, HC, et al. Parenteral glutamine dipeptide supplementation does not ameliorate chemotherapy-induced toxicity. Cancer 1994;74:2879-2884.

379. Vandenbroucke, JB. A short note on the history of the randomized controlled trial. J Chron Dis 1987;40:985-987.

380. Venook, AP. Bile duct. In: Dollinger, 1991:216-220.

381. Venook, AP. Liver. In: Dollinger, 1991:392-398.

382. Veronesi, A, et al. High-dose vs. low-dose cisplatin in advanced head and neck squamous carcinoma: a randomized study. JCO 1985;3:1105-1108.

383. Von Hoff, DD, et al., 'Single' agent activity of high-dose methotrexate with citrovorum factor rescue. Cancer Treat Rep 1978;62:233-235.

384. Von Hoff, DD, et al. Risk factors for doxorubicin-induced congestive heart failure. Ann Int Med 1979;91:710-717.

385. Vorherr, H. Adjuvant chemotherapy of breast cancer: hope—reality—hazard? Klin Wochenschr 1984;62:149-161.

386. Waksman, S and Woodruff, HB. Bacteriostatic and bacteriocidal substances produced by a soil actinomyces. Proc Soc Exper Biol & Med 1940;45:609.

387. Wang, J, et al. Enhancing effect of anti-tumor polysaccharide from astragalus or radix hedysarum on C3 cleavage production of macrophages in mice. Jpn J Pharmacol 1989;51:432-434.

388. Wangensteen, OH. Unconditionally yes. In: Standard, S and Nathan, H. Should the patient know the truth? NY: Springer, 1955:72-78.

389. Ward, PS. The American reception of salvarsan. JHMAS 1981:36.

390. Weiss, R and Muggia, F. Cytotoxic drug-induced pulmonary disease: update 1980. Amer J Med 1980;68:259-266.

391. Wiernik, PH, et al. Phase I trial of taxol given as a 24-hour infusion every 21 days: responses observed in metastatic melanoma. JCO 1987;5:1232-1239.

REFERENCES

392. Wilbur, DW, et al. Chemotherapy of non-small-cell lung carcinoma guided by an in vitro drug resistance assay measuring total tumour cell kill. Br J Cancer 1992;65:27-32.

393. Wilcox, PM, et al. Anticipatory vomiting in women receiving cyclophosphamide, methotrexate and 5-FU (CMF) adjuvant chemotherapy for breast carcinoma. Cancer Treat Rep 1982;66:1601-1604.

394. Wilson, AJ, et al. Adjuvant therapy for breast cancer. In: Slevin and Staquet, 1986: 359-383.

395. Wittes, RE and Hubbard, S. Chemotherapy: the properties and uses of single agents. In: Wittes, 1991: 66-121.

396. Wittes, RE. [ed.] Manual of oncologic therapeutics 1991/1992. Philadelphia: J.B. Lippincott, 1991.

397. Wolf, GT, et al. Induction chemotherapy for organ preservation in advanced squamous cell carcinoma of the oral cavity and oropharynx. Recent Results Cancer Res 1994;134:133-143.

398. Wright, JG, et al. Ask patients what they want. Evaluation of individual complaints before total hip replacement. J Bone Joint Surg Br 1994;76:229-234.

399. Yagoda, A. Bladder; kidney; and testis. In: Dollinger, 1991.

400. Young, LS, et al. Patients receiving glutamine-supplemented intravenous feedings report an improvement in mood. J Parenter Enteral Nutr 1993;17:422-427.

401. Zacharski, LR, et al. The biological basis for anticoagulant treatment for cancer. In: Jamieson, GA. Interaction of platelets and tumour cells. NY: Alan J. Liss, 1984:113-127.

402. Zhang, ZL, et al. Hepatoprotective effects of astragalus root. J Ethnopharmacol 1990;30:145-149.

403. Zheng, RY, et al. [Relationship between levamisole and encephalitis syndrome.] Chung-Hua Nei Ko Tsa Chih 1992;31:530-532.

404. Ziegler, TR, et al. Clinical and metabolic efficacy of glutamine-supplemented parenteral nutrition after bone marrow transplantation. A randomized, double-blind, controlled study. Ann Intern Med 1992;116:821-828.

405. Ziegler, TR. Glutamine is essential for epidermal growth factor-stimulated intestinal cell proliferation. J Parenter Enteral Nutr 1994;18:84-86.

406. Zinner, NR. Prostate. In: Dollinger, 1991:485-495.

407. Zoubek, A, et al. Ondansetron in the control of chemotherapy-induced and radiotherapy-induced emesis in children with malignancies. Anticancer Drugs 1993;4:Suppl 2:17-21.

408. Zubrod, CG. Chemical control of cancer [based on a National Academy of Sciences symposium held in October, 1991]. PNAS 1972;69:1042-1046.

Index

Abel, Ulrich, 32, 41, 48, 56, 59, 64-65, 73, 94, 96, 109, 113, 134, 151-153
ABV regimen, 124, 171
ABVD regimen, 128, 185
Acadia Institute, 55
Aches, 141, 185
ACTH, 19
Acupuncture, 168
Adenocarcinoma, 8, 107, 134-135, 142, 149, 177
Adenosquamous, 135
Adjuvants, 8, 14, 51, 53-54, 82, 84-94, 100-103, 107-108, 118, 120, 123, 131, 141, 146-149, 163
Adrenals, 115-116, 143, 175, 186
Adriamycin, 76, 156-157, 171, 181
Africa, 9
African-American, 143
Aging, 10, 139
AHCPR, 77
AIDS, 124
Alexander, Peter, 16
Alkeran, 171, 174
Alkylating agents, 15, 18, 70, 126, 132-133, 173-177, 185
Allopurinol, 127, 17
Aloe vahombe, 160
Aloe vera, 159-160
Altman, Lawrence K., 22, 27
Altretamine, 171-173, 185
American Cancer Society, 20, 26, 38, 65, 73, 77, 89, 93, 139
Amgen, 64, 76
Aminopterin, 177
AML, 126, 180-181
Amsacrine, 127
Anderson, M.D., 21, 132, 137
Anemia, 183
Anesthetics, 94
Angier, Natalie, 24
Annas, George, 154
Anorexia, 93, 116, 179-180, 183
Antabuse, 187
Anti-emetics, 76, 156
Anti-oxidants, 157
Anti-ulcer, 136
Antibiotic, 70, 127, 173, 177, 180, 183
Antibodies, 12, 15, 133
Anticoagulants, 161
Anticonvulsant, 186
Antiemetics, 177
Antiestrogen, 138
Antigens, 138-139
Antihistamines, 190
Antimetabolites, 19, 125, 158, 173, 177, 185
Antioxidants, 134, 157-158
Antman, Karen, 58
Anus, 116, 179, 183
Anxiety, 26, 36, 65, 151
Ara-C, 68, 171, 179
Armamentarium, 20, 22

Armpit, 18, 83, 89
Arms, 46, 48-49, 58, 128, 131
Arrhythmia, 184
Arsenic, 15
Arteries, 130
Arthralgias, 102
Asbestos, 132
Ascites, 115
Asia, 122, 159-160
Asparaginase, 171, 187
Aspergillosis, 69
Aspirin, 45, 161, 179
Astrocytomas, 118-120
Austin, Steve, 85, 90, 93, 158
Australia, 148
Austria, 99
AZT, 124

BACON regimen, 172
BACOP regimen, 172
Bacteria, 21, 45, 69, 179-180
Bailar, John, 31-32, 34
Bananas, 187
Barbiturates, 182, 186
Basal cell cancers (BCC), 141
Basiloid carcinomas, 183
BCG vaccine, 131
BCNU, 27, 35, 70, 171, 176
Benzene, 15
Beta-carotene, 157-158
BiCNU, 171, 176
Bile and biliary, 116, 130
Bioflavonoids, 158
Biohazards, 67-68
Biometry, 32
Biopsies, 147, 149
Biostatistician, 32, 34, 41, 54, 86
Biostatistics, 22, 31, 60, 86
Bladder, 12, 57, 78, 117-118, 137, 160, 164, 176-177, 182, 184-185, 189
Bladder-protecting agents, 106
Blenoxane, 171, 181
Bleomycin, 121, 123-124, 137, 146, 161, 171-172, 181, 188
Blood, 12, 16, 18, 20, 27, 69, 93-94, 102, 106, 108, 118, 125-127, 129-130, 133, 136, 143, 156, 175-178, 181-190
Blood-brain barrier, 119
Blood-producing cells, 16, 94, 175, 182-183
BMT, 58, 74-75, 98, 144, 157
Bobst, Elmer, 26
Bolus injection, 132, 179
Bonadonna, Gianni, 88, 93
Bone, 5, 12, 16-18, 20, 58, 72, 74-75, 83, 88, 94, 98, 109-110, 114, 116, 118, 120, 125, 127, 129, 131-133, 140, 144, 157, 159, 164, 175-176, 179-180, 184, 186, 188
Bone marrow depression, 16, 175, 179

Bowel, 53, 86, 116, 142, 188
Bowel-tolerance limit, 157
Boyle, Robert, 53
BPH, 137
Bradycardia, 156
Brain, 11, 69, 118-121, 126, 130, 137, 176, 178, 180, 184-187
Brandeis, Hon. Louis, 168
Braverman, Albert, 8-9, 20, 33, 59
Breast, 6, 8, 11-12, 14-16, 21, 24, 31, 35-36, 51-54, 56-58, 60-61, 69, 71, 73-74, 78, 82-92, 94-95, 97-98, 107, 128, 140, 149, 155, 164, 174-175, 177-179, 182-183, 185, 188, 190-191
Bristol-Myers Squibb, 69, 76, 79, 171
British, 8, 16, 45, 51, 87-88, 92, 94, 97, 99, 117-118, 161
Broder, Samuel, 51
Bromocriptine, 137
Bronchus, 50
Bross, Irwin, 22-23, 32-34, 54, 86-87
Burger, Hon. Warren, 168
Burkitt's lymphoma, 8, 27, 81
Burroughs-Wellcome, 76, 171
Busulfan, 70, 126-127, 171, 175
Buzhong yiqi, 160

C-MOPP, 129
Cachexia, 11
Cairns, John, 28-29, 31-32, 47, 50, 81, 122, 139-140
Calcium, 136, 179, 184
Calomel, 20, 72
Cameron, Charles, 20
CAMP, 110, 154, 172
Canada, 9, 40-42, 50-53, 131, 144, 173
Carboplatin, 69, 74, 112, 114, 127, 148-149, 160, 171, 176, 184-185
Carcinogens, 70, 163, 174, 180, 186
Carcinoid, 142, 147, 177
Cardiotoxicity, 69, 157, 177, 186
Cardozo, Hon. Benjamin, 168
Carmustine, 70, 117, 119, 124, 142, 171, 176
Carotenoids, 134, 157-158
Cartilage, 12, 140
Cataracts, 175
CCNU, 106, 108, 135, 171, 176
CEA, 61
Cerubidine, 171, 181
Cervix, 12, 49, 120, 148, 181-185
Cesium implants, 149
Chabner, Bruce, 22, 185, 187
Charlatanism, 16, 38, 41, 43
Chemo-embolization, 130
Chemotherapists, 9, 14-23, 27, 34, 40, 43, 53, 56-57, 112, 121, 135, 143, 146, 152, 187

Chest, 83, 105, 110, 128, 132, 144, 147
Chicago Tribune, 24, 53-54
Childhood cancer, 5, 9, 19-21, 28, 71, 119, 125-126, 129, 140, 142-143, 163, 178, 188
Children, 6, 12, 27-28, 44, 49, 58, 68, 75, 93, 115, 125-126, 129, 140, 142-144, 156, 174, 183, 187
Chile, 9, 144
Chills, 142, 181
China, 82, 102, 159-160
Chlebowski, Rowan, 102
Chlorambucil, 113, 127, 171, 175
Chloramphenicol, 176
Chlorpromazine, 176
Cholecystectomy, 122
Chondrosarcoma, 140
CHOP, 22, 129, 172
Choriocarcinoma, 8, 28, 81, 121-122, 146, 178, 183, 188
Choroid plexus carcinoma, 119
Circadian rhythms, 162
Cisplatin, 40, 74, 78, 109-110, 112-115, 117-119, 122-123, 132, 137, 143-144, 146-150, 156, 160, 162, 171-172, 179, 184-185
CLL, 127, 175
Clusters of cancer cases, 143
CMF, 85, 88, 90, 93-94, 96, 172, 175
CMFP, 90, 172
CMFVP, 95, 172
CML, 127
CNS, 69, 118, 176
Colon, 6, 12-14, 43-44, 61, 73, 82, 99-103, 142, 163, 179
Colorectal, 99-103, 137, 140, 182
Coma, 69, 178-180, 187
Constipation, 126, 155, 185-186, 188
Cooper regimen (CMFVP), 95
COP, 22, 172
COP-BLAM, 22, 172
Corticosteroids, 190
Cortisone, 19
Corynebacteria, 128
Cosmegen, 170, 183
Costs, 46, 74, 77-79, 90-91, 93, 103, 110, 112, 131, 154, 159, 175-176, 179-182, 186
Cost-benefit analysis, 78
Cuba, 148
Cyclophosphamide, 22, 27, 69-72, 78, 81, 88, 105, 108-110, 112, 117, 119-120, 126-127, 132, 136-137, 140, 143-144, 147-148, 150, 157, 160-161, 170-176, 179, 183, 188
Cyclosporine, 174
Cystadenocarcinomas, 135
Cystectomy, 118
Cysteine, 158
Cystitis, 106
Cytarabine, 68, 119, 126, 170-171, 179-180
Cytosar-U, 171, 179
Cytidine, 133
Cytokines, 7, 76
Cytoxan, 171, 175

CYVADIC, 141, 171
Czechoslovakia, 99, 104, 125

Dacarbazine, 131, 136, 140-141, 150, 171-172, 185, 188
Dactinomycin, 81, 121, 141, 143, 171-172, 180, 183
Dana-Farber Institute, 22
Dao, Thomas, 31, 87
Daunorubicin, 47, 126, 171, 180-182
DDT, 116, 137, 186
De-wormer, 101, 103
Denmark, 9, 82, 99, 125
Depression, 151, 186
DES, 138
DeVita, Vincent, 34, 46, 70, 73, 95, 119, 128, 162
Dexamethasone, 172
Diarrhea, 25, 93, 102, 116, 126, 157, 178-180, 183, 185-187, 190
Digoxin, 176, 180-182
Dilantin, 176, 180-182
Discoloration, 176, 181-182
Dizziness, 102, 177
DNA, 61, 141, 173, 175, 177, 180-184, 188
Dollinger, Malin, 116, 124, 145
Double-blind test, 46-47, 159
Dougherty, Thomas, 17
Doxorubicin, 70, 72, 78, 108-110, 112, 117-118, 121, 124, 126, 130, 132-133, 136, 140-141, 143-144, 147-148, 157, 162, 171-172, 179, 181-183, 185, 188
DTIC-Dome, 171, 185
Duke, Cuthbert E., 67, 94, 100
Dutch, 113, 159
Dyscrasia, 125

Ear, 6, 69, 184
Economics, 55, 76, 78, 80, 98
Ecuador, 99, 104, 148
Efudex, 179
Ehrlich, Paul, 15
Elspar, 171, 187
Emesis, 25, 156
Emodin, 160
Encephalitis, 102
Encephalopathies, 126
Endicott, Kenneth, 20-21
Endometrium, 148-149
Endoxan, 176
England, 29, 31, 39, 53-54, 60-61, 82, 87, 89-90, 138
Enteritis, 69
Enzymes, 135, 177-179, 184, 187
EORTC, 45, 55-56, 85-86, 88, 94-95, 97, 105, 108, 112, 119, 131
Ependymoma, 119
Epidemiology, 31-32, 49, 70, 128, 140, 152,
Epipodophyllotoxins, 187, 189
Epitheliomas, 12, 129
Epithelium, 17
Epstein, Samuel S., 30
Epstein-Barr virus, 128
Erythema, 181
Esophagus, 12, 122, 142, 179
Estramustine, 138

Estrogens, 84, 119, 148
Etoposide, 69, 74, 78, 119, 127, 136, 141, 146, 171-172, 177, 189-190
Eulexin, 138
Europe, 38, 87, 187
Europeans, 45, 56, 85-86, 95, 97, 105, 119, 131, 191
Ewing sarcoma, 8, 28, 81, 140, 183, 188-189
Extravasation, 174, 181, 188
Extremities, 69, 131
Eyes, 6, 31, 33, 37, 59, 137, 114, 144, 167, 176

Face, 34, 67, 185
Fats, 99
Fear, 8, 25-26, 36
Feinstein, Alvan, 50, 60-62, 123, 152
Fetus, 121-122, 130, 143, 174, 186
Fever, 142, 181, 185
Fibrosis, 178
FIGO, 13, 112, 114
Filgrastim, 7, 118, 155
Fingernails, 182
Fingertips, 181
Finsen Institute (Copenhagen), 41, 106
Fisher, Bernard, 54, 86, 90
Fludarabine, 127
Fluoropyrimidines, 179
Fluorouracil, 27, 88, 90, 100, 101, 116-117, 119, 122, 133, 136, 141, 149, 157, 159, 161-162, 171-172, 177, 179
Flutamide, 138
Folic acid, 156, 158, 177-178
Folinic acid (leucovorin), 178
Food and Drug Administration (FDA), 8-9, 45, 66, 67, 72, 74, 79, 115, 191
Foxglove, 161
France, 9, 133
Fraud, 3, 24, 43, 53-55, 57, 59, 61, 63, 65, 86
French, 20, 34, 36, 128, 191
Frost & Sullivan, 75-76
Ftorafur, 179
FUDR, 179
Fungi, 69, 183
Fungoides, 57, 188

Gall bladder, 122
Gastric, 20, 73, 136, 144-145
Gastrointestinal, 17, 116, 142, 175, 179-180, 183, 186
Genetics, 13, 79, 99, 143, 173, 180-181, 184
Genitals, 148
Germany, 9, 32, 40-41, 82, 95-99, 125, 151, 157, 161, 175, 177
Gestational tumors, 121
Ginseng, 161
Glands, 116, 135-138, 144, 147, 175-176, 178, 181, 186
Glaxo, Inc., 25, 64, 76-77
Glioblastoma, 118-120
Glioma, 119-120
Glutamine, 159
Glutathione, 158

Granulocytes, 75, 182
Granulocytopenia, 102
Great Britain, 9, 45, 151
Greece, 133
Greenberg, Daniel, 26, 29-30

Hair, 20, 39, 67, 93, 106, 114,
  157, 174-175, 179, 181-183,
  186, 188, 190
Hallucinations, 176, 185
Haloperidol, 176
Halsted mastectomy, 85, 89
Hansen, Heine H., 41
Haskell, Charles, 110-111
Head, 12, 14, 18, 25, 31, 54, 57,
  87, 120, 122-123, 152, 178-179,
  181, 183-186
Headaches, 25, 45, 93, 102, 142,
  155, 177, 186-187
Heart, 22, 79, 118, 156-157,
  175-176, 181-182, 190
Hematology, 22, 33, 67
Hemolyticuremic, 183
Hemorrhages, 106, 187
Hepatitis, 188
Herbs, 43, 159-161, 187
Hexalen, 171, 173, 185
Hexamethylmelamine, 185
Hill, Austin, 45
Hitchcock, Kathy, 85, 90, 93, 114
HIV, 124
Hives, 177, 186-187
Hodgkin's disease, 5, 8-9, 12,
  20-21, 27-28, 39, 70-72, 81,
  124, 127-129, 163, 177, 182,
  185-186, 188-189
Hormonal treatment, 19, 76, 83,
  92, 95-96, 137-138, 163, 173
Hormones, 71, 84, 87, 95, 116,
  126, 136, 138-139, 148, 184,
  186
Hospices, 50, 74
Hungary, 99, 104, 125, 133
Hunter, John, 84-85
Hydatidiform, 121
Hydrazine sulfate, 161
Hydrea, 171, 186
Hydroxyurea, 119, 121, 125,
  127, 171, 186
Hypercalcemia, 136, 184
Hyperplasia, 137, 149
Hypersensitivity, 115, 190
Hypertensive, 187
Hyperthermia, 131
Hypnotic, 186

ICE, 22, 69, 149, 172-176, 189
Iceland, 148
Idamycin, 171, 182
Idarubicin, 171, 182
IFEX, 69, 171, 176
Ifosfamide, 69, 74, 106, 140-141,
  171-172, 176
Ihde, Daniel, 105-106
Immunostimulants, 103, 131
Immunosuppressants, 160, 174,
  186
Immunotherapy, 101-102,
  131-133
Infants, 142-143
Infections, 21, 45, 69, 109, 124,
  128, 159, 180, 190

Inflammation, 141, 174, 176,
  178, 183-184, 190
Insecticide, 116, 137, 186
Insomnia, 102
Insulin, 45
Insulinomas, 136
Interferons, 74, 76, 122, 124,
  127, 133, 141-142
Interleukins, 76, 154, 157
Intestinal, 99, 102, 142, 159, 176
Ireland, 82, 99
Israel, 20-21, 34, 36, 125
Italy, 9, 16, 88, 121, 125
Itching, 181
Japan, 38-39, 82, 111, 137, 144,
  160
Jaundice, 175, 180
Juzen-taiho-to, 161
Jönsson, Bengt, 78-79

Kampo medicine, 160
Kaposi's sarcoma, 124, 140, 188
Karnofsky, David, 19, 120
Karolinska Institute, 148
Kefauver-Harris Amend., 45
Kidneys, 69, 114, 109, 116, 118,
  124-125, 143, 160, 174,
  176-178, 182-1845, 186
Kotlowitz, Robert, 36-37, 68
Kushner, Rose, 89, 92
L-asparaginase, 126
L-PAM, 87-88, 156, 171
Lactobacilli, 161
Larynx, 123, 152, 181
Laszlo, John, 93-94
Leibovitz, Brian, 158
Lejeune, Ferdy, 131
Leucovorin rescue factor, 90,
  104, 133, 140, 142, 172, 178
Leukemia, 5, 8-9, 15, 19-21, 25,
  27-28, 49, 57, 70-71, 75, 78, 81,
  125-128, 133, 140, 164, 175,
  178, 180-182, 184, 188
Leukeran, 171, 175
Leukocytes, 12, 125
Leukopenia, 143, 186
Leuprolide, 138
Levamisole, 100-103, 131, 164,
  179
Licorice, 161
Lilly, Eli, 171
Lithium carbonate, 161
Local tumors, 65, 85-86, 99,
  119-120, 132-133, 136, 138, 142
Lomustine, 70, 108, 110, 124,
  154, 171-172, 176
Lonidamine, 124-125
Lumpectomy, 84
Lung, 6, 8, 10-13, 24, 34, 36,
  40-42, 49-50, 56-57, 61-62,
  68-69, 73, 78-79, 82-83, 102,
  104-105, 107-108, 110, 112,
  135, 137, 150, 152-154, 160,
  164, 165, 174-176, 178,
  181-185, 187, 189-191
Luxembourg, 82, 134
Lycopene, 158
Lymph system, 12, 18, 83, 86,
  116, 122, 128-131, 138, 142,
  150, 161, 176, 178, 181
Lymphoblastic, 126
Lymphocytes, 12, 127, 133

Lymphocytic, 8, 27, 49, 57, 81,
  125-127, 164, 175, 180-181, 188
Lymphoid, 12, 16, 127, 129
Lymphoma, 5, 8, 11-12, 17, 28,
  69, 72, 81, 120, 124, 127, 129,
  135, 142, 147-148, 175-176,
  178, 182, 185, 188-189
Lymphosarcoma, 8, 17, 28, 81
Lysodren, 116, 171, 186

M-BACOD, 129, 172
MACC, 108, 172
Macroglobulinemia, 175
Maculopapular rash, 186-187
Madagascar, 160
Magnesium, 179
Malformations, 143, 174, 186
Mammography, 31, 60-61
Marrow, bone, 16-18, 20, 58,
  74-75, 88, 94, 98, 109-110, 114,
  118, 120, 125, 127, 129, 131-
  133, 144, 157, 159, 165, 175-
  176, 179-180, 184, 186, 188
Mastectomy, 85, 88-89, 94
Matulane, 161, 171, 186
Mauritius, 148
Mayapple, 187-188
Mayo Clinic, 74, 101-103, 133, 145
Mechlorethamine, 171-172, 174
Medulloblastoma, 119-120, 147
Megace, 138
Melanocytes, 12
Melanoma, malignant, 10-13,
  103, 130-132, 136, 141, 149-
  150, 161, 174, 182, 185, 190
Melphalan, 70, 132-133, 171-175
Memorial Sloan-Kettering
  Cancer Center, 5-7, 16, 18, 22,
  30-31, 35, 79-80, 86, 160
Menadione, 157
Meningiomas, 120
Menopause, 84
Menstruation, 174-175
Mercaptopurine, 171, 180
Merck, Inc., 76, 171
Mesna, 106, 176
Mesothelioma, 132-133, 185
Meta-analyses, 63-64, 91
Metastases, 11-12, 14, 17, 61-62,
  66, 71, 83, 86, 97, 99, 117, 119,
  121-122, 150
Methotrexate, 27-28, 71-72, 78,
  81, 88, 90, 94, 108, 110, 117-
  118, 121, 133, 137, 140, 144,
  157-159, 171-172, 176-179,
  183, 188
Mexico, 49, 121
Micrometastases, 14, 84-86, 108
Misconduct, 55
Mithracin, 171, 184
Mitomycin, 117, 121-122, 137,
  149-150, 161, 171-172, 179, 183
Mitotane, 116, 137, 171, 186
Mitoxantrone, 47, 127, 148, 171,
  182
Miyaji, Naoko, 39
Moertel, Chas., 74, 101, 103, 145
Mole, 12, 121
Monoblastic leukemia, 126
Monocytic leukemia, 126
Mouth, 67, 133, 159, 176, 178,
  180, 183, 185-186, 188

INDEX

Mouth sores, 67, 159, 176, 178-180, 183, 185, 188
Mucositis, 69, 190
Mutamycin, 171, 183
Myeloblastic leukemia, 126, 188
Myelocytic leukemia, 175
Myelodysplastic, 125
Myelogenous leukemia, 126-127
Myeloid, 78, 126-127, 180-181
Myeloma, multiple, 10, 12, 57, 133, 161, 174-175, 188
Myelosuppression, 88, 95
Myleran, 171, 175

Nasopharynx, 123
National Cancer Data Base, 73-74, 83, 100, 103, 111, 144
Nausea, 47, 67-68, 76, 93, 102, 106, 109-110, 114, 126, 151, 155-157, 174-177, 189-190
National Cancer Institute, 5, 19-20, 26, 31, 34, 51-54, 57-58, 70-71, 73, 77, 84, 90, 98, 100-101, 103, 105-106, 119, 124, 131-132, 154, 157, 165-166, 177, 179, 184-185, 187
Neoadjuvants, 123
Neosar, 171, 176
Nephroblastoma, 1843
Nerves, 114, 137, 152, 156, 178, 184-185, 188-190
Netherlands, 104
Neupogen, 7, 118, 155
Neuroblastoma, 143, 188-189
Neuropathy, 110, 156, 185
Neurotoxicity, 95
Neutrophils, 191
New Zealand, 82, 99, 125, 137
Niacin, 156
Nicotinamide, 156
National Institutes of Health (NIH), 80, 86, 89, 91, 101, 165
Nitrogen mustard, 16-18, 27, 70-71, 171, 173-174, 177
Nitrosoureas, 70, 124, 176-177
Non-Hodgkin's lymphoma, 12, 69, 72, 129, 148, 175, 178, 182, 188-189
Norway, 97, 137
Novantrone, 171, 182
NSABP, 53-54, 86-87, 90, 93
NSCLC, 40, 49, 104, 107, 109, 153, 189, 191
Nursing, 22, 37, 47, 50, 67, 93, 175-176
Nutrition, 68, 157-159, 164, 170, 187

Octreotide, 136
Off-label usage, 9, 74, 189
Oncologists, 5, 13, 22, 25, 29, 35, 40-44, 53, 56, 59, 71, 74, 80, 87, 90, 92-96, 102, 110, 112, 114, 129, 151-155, 164-165, 177
Oncology, 3, 9, 22, 27, 33-35, 37, 39, 41-42, 57, 67, 69-70, 76, 84, 90, 101, 119
Oncotech, 162
Oncovin, 171, 188
Ondansetron, 25, 127, 155-156
Oral, 133-134, 156, 189
Orchiectomy, 146

Oropharynx, 123
Orthodox medicine, 40, 47, 57-59, 64, 70, 79, 132-133, 165
Osteosarcoma, 5, 140, 1789
Ovarian, 8, 12, 35, 57, 63-64, 69-70, 73, 82, 92, 111-115, 163, 174-175, 177, 184-186, 189-191

Paclitaxel, 68, 114-115, 132, 171, 173, 187, 189, 191
Palliation, 14, 32, 85, 99, 107, 112, 116, 119, 122-125, 141, 145, 151-153, 163-165, 186
Pancreas, 12, 34, 38, 73, 82, 134-135, 177, 179-180, 183-184
Paraneoplastic syndrome, 152
Paraplatin, 171, 184-185
Parasites, 188
Parathyroid, 136, 184
Pauling, Linus, 157
PDQ system, 84, 98, 100, 104, 132-133, 166
Pelvis, 144, 150
Penicillin, 19, 21, 45
Penis, 136-137, 181
Periwinkle, 187-188
Pfizer, Inc., 80
Phenylalanine, 174
Phlebitis, 190
Photosensitizers, 142
Physicians' Desk Ref., 47, 174
Pituitary, 137
Placebos, 46-48, 58, 86-87, 102, 105-106, 108, 156, 163, 165
Plant-derived drugs, 173, 187
Platelets, 176, 186
Platinol, 28, 109, 112-114, 160, 170-173, 184
Plicamycin, 171, 184
Pneumonia, 47, 181, 183
Pneumonitis, 178
Podophyllum, 188
Poland, 104
Prednisone, 70, 126-128, 133, 171, 181
Pregnancy, 28, 121, 146, 175-176
Premalignancies, 99, 126
Premenopausal women, 85-86, 88-89, 92, 94, 163
Premyelocytic, 126
Procarbazine, 70, 110, 119, 161, 170-171, 186-187
Profits, in chemotherapy, 6-7, 19, 42, 62, 76, 80, 154, 164
Prolactin, 137
Promace, 22, 171
Promace-cytabom, 72, 129
Prostate, 10, 57, 61, 137-140, 182
Prostatectomy, 138
Pseudo-leukemia, 128
Psoriasis, 179
Purinethol, 171, 180

Quackery, 16, 41, 164

Radiation, 14, 43, 65, 70, 73-75, 90, 92, 105-107, 109, 111-112, 116, 119-121, 123, 128-129, 134, 137-138, 140-141, 143-150, 152, 157, 160, 179-183
Radiotherapy, 28, 70, 78, 105, 110, 121-123, 128, 145-147, 157

Radner, Gilda, 114
Randomized Clinical (or Controlled) Trials, 43-46, 53, 57-58, 92, 110, 164
Rankin, Elaine, 49, 55, 105, 108, 110, 153
Rectal, 12, 73, 99-100, 140, 142, 179, 183
Recurrences, 14, 65, 84, 86-87, 91, 101, 104, 108, 143, 147, 149
Reed-Sternberg cells, 128
Relapses, 13-14, 28, 66, 71, 88, 90, 106, 116, 133, 143, 146, 183
Remissions, 11, 13-14, 19-20, 27-28, 43, 59, 65-66, 78, 104, 111-112, 114, 116, 120, 122, 128, 131, 145, 153, 180, 182, 185, 188
Renal, 110
Rescue factor, 25, 90, 104, 133, 140, 178
Retching, 5, 20
Retinoblastoma, 8, 28, 81, 144
Retinoids, 141, 157
Rhabdomyosarcoma, 8, 28, 81, 140, 183, 188
Rhoads, Cornelius, 18-21
Rhone-Poulenc, Inc., 191
Rights of patients, 164-168
RNA, 179-182, 184
Rosenbaum, Ernest, 145
Rosenberg, Steven, 132
Roswell Park, 22, 31, 33, 86-87
Russia, 159

Sacrum, 116
Salvarsan, 15
Sandostatin, 136
Sandoz, Inc., 76-77
Sarcoma, 5, 8, 28, 81, 124, 140, 148, 178, 183, 188-189
Sarcomas, 11-12, 136, 140-142, 149, 182, 185
Sarna, Gregory, 34
Scarring, 128, 175-176, 181
Schipper, Harvey, 23
Schmidt, Benno, 79
SCLC, 8, 104-107, 188
Scotland, 104
SEER, 49, 51, 105
Seizures, 126, 175, 178, 184, 186
Seminomas, 146
Semustine, 131, 179
Serum, 139, 187
Shapiro, Martin, 27, 34, 80, 111, 154, 165-166
Shimkin, Morris, 71
Simone, Charles, 90, 157
Singapore, 133, 148
Single-agent, 71, 107, 114, 135
Skin, 67, 83, 116, 130, 136, 141, 174-182, 184, 186, 188
Slevin, Maurice, 112
Small-cell, 8, 13, 57, 79, 82, 104-105, 160, 163, 185, 189
Smoking, 49-50, 104, 107
Solid tumors, 6, 8, 28, 63, 73, 81, 85, 129, 142, 146, 181, 183-186
Somatostatin, 136
Spain, 5, 64
Spasms, 179, 187
Sponges, 67, 94, 180

Spontaneous remissions, 11
Spread of disease, 11-12, 14, 27, 39, 43, 65, 71, 83, 85, 99-100, 105, 107, 116, 119, 121, 128, 130, 134-136, 138, 141, 144, 147, 149, 164
Squamous cell cancer, 107, 122, 136-137, 141, 149, 181
Stage-migration bias, 62
Staging, 12-13, 99, 116, 129
Statistics, 28-30, 31, 44-45, 49-52, 55, 60, 62-63, 83, 97, 100, 103, 123, 129, 139, 141, 154
Status, 33, 49, 109, 126, 152, 164
Sterility, 175
Stern, Jeffrey, 149
Steroids, 156, 176
Stomach, 12, 49, 57, 82, 122, 144-146, 179, 183
Streptomycin, 19, 45, 180
Streptozocin, 70, 136, 142, 170, 177
Stress, 116
Strokes, 126
Stupor, 188
Sugar, 46-47, 102, 156, 177, 188
Sugiura, Kanematsu, 4, 16
Sulfanilamide, 19, 21, 176
Sulfonamides, 19
Supplementation, 156-157, 159
Suramin, 139
Surgery, 8, 14, 24, 31, 43-44, 51, 55, 73, 78, 81-82, 84, 86-87, 89-90, 92, 99-102, 107-109, 111-112, 116, 118-120, 122-123, 130-131, 134-138, 140-149, 152, 156, 179, 183
Sweating, 187
Sweden, 78, 137, 148-149
Swelling, 119, 187
Switzerland, 95, 137
Syphilis, 15

Taiwan, 157
Tamoxifen, 78, 85, 90, 124-125, 148-150, 163, 171, 174
Taxol, 68, 114-115, 132, 171, 173, 187, 189-191
Taxotere, 191
Teniposide, 171, 189
Teratogenic, 186
Teratomas, 78, 146
Terminal (word), 11, 56
Testicular, 8, 12, 28, 78, 81, 109, 146, 163, 176, 181-185, 188-189
Texas, 97, 160
Thiamine, 156
Thiazide-type, 179
Thioguanine, 126, 171, 181-182
Thiotepa, 86-87, 132, 145, 171, 177
Thrombocytes, 190
Thrombocytopenia, 107, 186
Thrombophlebitis, 174
Thymolipomas, 147
Thymoma, 147
Thymus, 147
Thyroid, 136, 147-148, 182
TNM system, 12-13, 61, 99, 105, 116, 123
Tobacco, 50, 134

Tomato, 158-159
Tongue, 123
Tonics, 159
Tonsils, 123
Toxicity, 3, 18, 20, 34, 39-40, 48, 67-69, 71-72, 93-94, 102, 106-110, 112-116, 118, 124, 143, 146, 155-162, 163, 176-178, 180, 182, 184-187, 190
Toxicology, 2
Trachea, 12
Transfusions, 127
Transplantation, 17, 58, 74-75, 98, 127, 129, 131, 144, 157, 159
Tremors, 102
Trialists group, 91-92
Tromethamine, 179
Trophoblastic diseases, 121
Tuberculosis, 45, 128
Tyramine, 161, 187

University of California at Los Angeles, 34, 44, 165
Ulcers, 179
Upjohn, Inc., 76, 171
Uracil, 179
Ureter, 124
Urethral, 137
Uric acid, 127
Urinary, 117, 175, 178
Urination, 175, 186
Urine, 47, 106, 175, 181-184
Urologists, 106
Uruguay, 137
Uteri, cervix, 120, 148
Uterine, 120, 148-149, 182

Vaccines, 131
Vagina, 149-150
Vancouver, 39
Vascular, 71
Vegetables, 99, 134
Veins, 93, 105, 174, 190
Velban, 170, 188
Venereal disease, 15, 188
Venezuela, 148
Venook, Alan, 117, 130
Venous system, 174
Venture-capital, 6
Vepesid, 171, 188
Vertex, 79
Vesicant, 174
Vietnam, 23, 30
Vinblastine, 117, 124, 146, 171-172, 188
Vinca alkaloids, 187
Vincristine, 27, 68, 70, 119, 124, 126, 141, 143-144, 147, 149, 157, 171-172, 179, 181, 183, 187-188
Vindesine, 78
Viruses, 143
Vitamin B1, 99, 156
Vitamin B2, 99, 156
Vitamin B12, 156, 185
Vitamins, 134, 141, 156-158, 177-178, 185
VM-26, 189
Vomiting, 25, 39, 67, 76, 93-94, 102, 106, 109-110, 114, 116, 126, 155-156, 174-177,

179-186, 189-190
Vorherr, H., 88
Vulva, 149-150, 181
Vumon, 171, 189

Wait-and-see attitude, 47, 109, 146, 154
Waksman, Selman, 183
Wales, 82
Wangensteen, Owen, 38
Warfarin, 102, 186
Warts, 188
Washington Post, 38, 54
Watermelon, 159
Watson, James, 29
Weisenthal, Larry, 162
Wilms' tumor, 8, 28, 81, 143, 183, 188
Wilson, Alan, 55, 85, 88, 92
Wittes, Robert, 5
Woburn, MA, 143
Womb, 120
Wounds, 125, 174
Wyeth-Ayerst, Inc., 171

X-rays, 43

Yagoda, Alan, 117-118, 124, 146
Yale University, 16-18, 50, 60, 62, 123, 152
Yew tree, 189-191
Yogurt, 161, 187
Yolk-sac tumor, 146

Zanosar, 171, 177
Zeneca, 64
Zidovudine (AZT), 124
Zinc, 15
Zinner, Norman, 138
Zofran (ondansetron), 25, 127, 155
Zubrod, Gordon, 81
Zyloprim (allopurinol), 127